Take Back Your Marriage

Take Back Your Marriage

SECOND EDITION

Sticking Together in a World
That Pulls Us Apart

WILLIAM J. DOHERTY, PhD

THE GUILFORD PRESS
New York   London

Published by The Guilford Press
A Division of Guilford Publications, Inc.
370 Seventh Avenue, Suite 1200, New York, NY 10001
www.guilford.com

Library of Congress Cataloging-in-Publication Data

Doherty, William J. (William Joseph), 1945–
  Take back your marriage : sticking together in a world that pulls
us apart / William J. Doherty. — Second edition.
    pages cm
  Includes index.
  ISBN 978-1-4625-0367-4 (pbk. : alk. paper) —
ISBN 978-1-4625-1046-7 (hardcover : alk. paper)
  1. Marriage. 2. Commitment (Psychology) I. Title.
  HQ734.D66 2013
  306.81—dc23

                                        2013006304

Part of the poem "Do Not Go Gentle into That Good Night" is reprinted
from *The Poems of Dylan Thomas*, copyright © 1952 by Dylan Thomas.
Reprinted by permission of New Directions Publishing Corp.

For Leah, still the one

Contents

Introduction

I began the first edition of this book with the story of a wedding I witnessed in the Plaza at Santa Fe, New Mexico, in 2000. As I was preparing this revision eleven years later, I came upon a wedding taking place while I was visiting St. Severin, an ancient church in Paris. This was a bilingual wedding, with parts recited in the groom's French and others in the bride's American English. But in most ways it was quite familiar: the wedding march music, the common biblical readings, the overlong sermon, the soloist enthusiastic but a bit flat, the bride and groom expectant and nervous. I settled in at the back row to enjoy the ritual while trying to make out the French words.

But as the bride recited her wedding vow, I sat up in my seat. I saw the guests stir as well. The vow started with the standard promise of personal love and commitment, but this bride had a bigger picture of marriage. She committed herself to having children together and launching a family that would reach through generations in time and impact. This was more than building a private life with her husband. Rather, this vow showed they were creating something that would stretch far beyond their own lifetimes. Suddenly the stakes were higher for this new marriage, the arc much longer. This many-generations vow made me recall the overwhelming moment when I learned of the birth of my first grandchild six years before. I pictured him, with good luck and improved health care, as living into the twenty-second century. I decided that if my job as a parent had been to prepare my children for the world, my job as a grandparent is to prepare the world for my grandchildren. The arc of a marriage, like that of parenting, is very long.

For me, a striking aspect of the bride's vows was that she was the American partner, not the European one. (I couldn't make out all of the groom's vows in French, so can't report what he said.) Europeans generally have been more focused on the solidarity between past and future generations, and many young Europeans get married only when they decide to have children. Americans approach marriage mostly as a love union for the couple; children are rarely mentioned in marriage vows. Not coincidentally, divorce is considerably higher in the United States than in countries like France. The sociologist Andrew Cherlin refers to the "marriage-go-round" in the United States in comparison to Western Europe. He notes that we have higher values and expectations of marriage as a union of soul mates, but deliver lower rates of stable marriages and families.

Some people argue that the way to resolve this contradiction between our values for lifelong marriage and our divorce rate is to change our values. One book for people considering divorce referred to "the obsolete mythology of love." The foremost myth about marriage, the falsehood most worthy of debunking, the author claimed, was "the myth of forever." The truth is that marriages end, the author observed. Holding onto the myth of permanence creates unnecessary crises in self-esteem when the marriage ends. The logic seems to be that lowering your expectations going in the front door will decrease your pain going out the back door. This is probably true, but notice the lack of any sense of the consequences for others beyond the couple. No sense here of generations to come.

Psychiatrist and prominent Fox TV commentator Keith Ablow would view that marriage counselor as being too optimistic about marriage. "The vast, vast majority of men and women," Ablow writes, "are no longer physically attracted to their spouses after five or ten years (that's being kind), if they have seen one another most of that time. Human beings just are not built to desire one another once we have flossed in the same room a hundred times and shared a laundry basket for thousands of days. . . . Marriage is a dying institution because it inherently deprives men and women of the joy of being 'chosen' on a daily basis."

New Jersey wedding consultant Sharon Naylor notes that she hears in wedding vows a lot of promises to be together "as long as our love shall last." "I personally think it's quite a statement on today's times—people know the odds of divorce," she says, adding that the rephrasing is part of a more general trend toward personalizing vows. Naylor said killing the "death vow" doesn't mean that people don't take their marriage promises seriously. Quite the contrary. "People understand that anything can happen in life, and you don't make a promise you can't keep. When people get divorced, they mourn the fact that they said ''til death do us part'—you didn't keep your word in church (if they had a church wedding). Some people are in therapy because they promised ''til death do us part'—it is the sticking point in the healing of a broken marriage. The wording can give you a stigma of personal failure." For those who have expressed interest in eliminating "'til death do us part," Naylor has suggested going with "For as long as our marriage shall serve the greatest good." "You will promise to be loyal as long as love shall last—you don't want to promise 'when you treat me like crap,'" she said.

For good reasons that I will explain, most of us want something more than a commitment for the foreseeable future. And our children certainly want more out of our unions. Let me be clear that I am not for any couple to get married if they are not ready for marriage or interested in it. Feeling forced into marriage could be a disaster for these couples. Nor am I prescribing marriage for every couple who are cohabiting but have already made a permanent commitment to each other and told the world about it. Americans don't respond well to being told what to do with their personal lives. I am more concerned about the new cultural pessimism about the possibility of permanent commitment in marriage, and how this pessimism, fueled by the consumer culture, by high divorce rates, and by some professional experts, is undermining the prospects for permanent commitment in marriage.

Sadly, this undermining seems to be mostly affecting people who could benefit greatly from stable marriages in an uncertain world. Over the past two decades, demographers have documented a growing marriage gap between college-educated couples and couples with less education. College-educated couples are experiencing lower divorce rates while other groups continue to have historically high rates. What's more, college-educated couples are following a life trajectory that leads to the best outcomes for adults and children in American society: they finish their education, then marry, then have children, and then stay married while raising their children. Working-class and low-income couples across the racial and ethnic groups are far more apt to have riskier trajectories: interrupted education, children before marriage, not marrying at all, or marrying and divorcing.

Sociologists like Kathryn Edin have shown how low-income, urban women and men still aspire to stable marriage but are skeptical that they can pull it off; they see marriage as the sweet but elusive icing on the cake after they achieve a middle-class lifestyle and find a sexually faithful partner. Marriage is not so much part of the journey but a destination at the end of a journey that already includes children and multiple cohabiting partners and breakups.

Given these trends, I worry that healthy, lifelong marriage is becoming another privilege of those with lots of resources in American culture. Children don't get to choose the couple who conceive them and the environment that either supports or undermines the ability of their parents to love, honor, and cherish each other—or to move on down the road. We have to believe in something more than our own relationships if lifelong, flourishing marriage is to be widely available to future generations. It's like a commitment to good education or health care: it's not enough to support health care and schooling for one's own family; we have to support opportunities for everyone or our own family will suffer the consequences, perhaps not immediately, but in future generations.

Because everything I say in this book hangs on the value of lifelong commitment, I will make the case here for its value. For starters, there is no question that most of us still desire a lifelong marriage commitment. If you are married, chances are that you pledged to stay married as long as you both shall live, and that you meant it. If you hope to be married some day, chances are that you plan to recite a similar pledge. Polls of young people show two things: that most still want a permanent marital commitment some day but are becoming skeptical that it's possible in today's world. The longing is still there, but the worries are greater than in any previous generation ever studied.

Why the pessimism about long-term commitment? Partly it's because of the historically high divorce rates. The younger generation has lived through their parents' experiments with marriage and divorce. Partly it's because of the growing skepticism of therapists and other professionals who have to work every day with what is real, not necessarily with what is ideal. Marriages come and go, many of my colleagues say, so let's accept that fact and make the best of it, rather than being nostalgic for an era of stable marriages that had their own dark sides. As one prominent family therapist used to say, speaking of his goals for couples, "The good marriage, the good divorce—it matters not." A sign of a cultural shift is that now he does not view his goals that way any longer, just as the minister who invented the marriage vow "as long as we both shall love" has recanted.

Family sociologists point out that the divorce rate goes up in every nation where women become educated and achieve economic independence. Let's accept the inevitability, they say, that many people will opt for divorce when they are not happy in their marriage and that many other people will avoid marriage by living together. The important thing is healthy, supportive "relationships," whether or not these are marriage relationships intended to last a lifetime.

This skeptical view of permanent marital commitment has much going for it, because it seems to fit the realities of our time. And it underlines the variety of choices now available for mating. But ultimately, it betrays our deepest longings for stable intimate bonds. It surrenders us to the "me-first" consumer culture in which keeping one's options open is seen as the key to success in life. Loyalty and permanent commitments are on the decline everywhere, from athletes to their teams and teams to their cities, from companies to their employees and employees to their companies. Why would we expect marriage to escape the pattern?

In fact, the idea of permanent commitment runs counter to everything we know about a market-based world, and especially the technology-driven, dot.com world we now live in. Success in today's turbomarket economy requires a mind-set that is the opposite of long-term commitments. It requires ruthlessness in shedding what no longer meets current needs and desires. The old must give way when it is no longer useful. The factories that made slide rules had to close when calculators became common. Community banks are gobbled up by conglomerates or they wither and die. When a national video store company misses the window to get into Internet delivery of movies, bankruptcy soon follows. Is it surprising that the nation that leads the world in forging the new economy also leads the world in divorce?

The irony is that many experts and some sophisticated couples are giving up on permanent marriage at the very time when the scientific research is showing us that this kind of relationship is good for us. Of course some marriages are destructive, but the evidence now is overwhelming that married people are healthier physically and psychologically, live longer, have more money, have fewer bad habits like smoking and excessive drinking, and are overall happier. Demographer Linda Waite and sociologist Paul Amato, among others, have summarized this research, including studies that have followed large groups of people from before marriage to after getting married. This research makes it clear that marriage confers important benefits on individuals, benefits that increase over the years, and not just that healthier people are the ones who get married in the first place. These benefits occur for both men and women, contrary to the popular misconception that marriage benefits men but not women.

And these are just the benefits for adults. Research has demonstrated convincingly what most people have known all along: that a stable, loving, two-parent family is the optimal environment for children's health and development in our society. The only dispute is whether children are better off when a failed marriage ends in divorce or the parents stay together. The most recent studies on this subject, surveying large numbers of families followed over many years, indicate that children do better when their unhappily married parents stay together as long as the parents do not engage in high levels of conflict. In Paul Amato and Alan Booth's major book-length study, *A Generation at Risk,* seventy percent of the marriages that ended were low-conflict relationships; in these cases, children on average did much more poorly than if their dissatisfied but low-conflict parents stayed together. In the thirty percent of high-conflict marriages, the children did better after the divorce. Other studies are pointing to the same conclusion—that children do better in homes with stable marriages as long as the parents are reasonably cooperative.

Although statistical averages do not reflect every individual experience, and no one should be expected to stay with an abusive or irresponsible spouse who won't change, the research is now compelling on the benefits of sustained marriage commitment. And these same benefits do not show up in cohabiting couples, except for cohabiting couples who are engaged to be married. The skeptics may be correct that this permanent marital commitment is difficult, but they are wrong in suggesting that most people are just as well off in other kinds of relationships. Marriage matters greatly.

Beyond what the research tells us, permanent commitment in marriage may be even more important in today's fragmented world than it ever was. Most of us do not dwell in lifelong communities where we can count on friends and neighbors being there decade after decade. Many of our grown children scatter around the continent or the world. Our siblings do the same. One of the first benefits I discovered about being married was the freedom to plan a long-term future with my wife. The marital horizon extends to the edge of our vision in a way that no other relationship does. And this allows for a degree of emotional safety to be fully ourselves, to struggle more openly than with anyone else in our lives, and to know another person more fully and deeply than is possible any other way.

Marriage with the long view comes with the conviction that nothing will break us up, that we will fight through whatever obstacles get in our way, that if the boat gets swamped we will bail it out, that we will recalibrate our individual goals if they get out of alignment, that we will share leadership for maintaining and renewing our marriage, that we will renovate our marriage if the current version gets stale, that if we fight too much or too poorly we will learn to fight better, that if sex is no longer good we will find a way to make it good again, that we will accept each other's weaknesses that can't be fixed, and that we will take care of each other in our old age. This kind of commitment is not made just once, but over and over through the course of a lifetime. We cling to it during the dark nights of the soul that come to nearly every marriage, times when the love is hard to feel but the promise keeps us together. The playwright Thornton Wilder said it well:

> I didn't marry you because you were perfect. I didn't even marry you because I loved you. I married you because you gave me a promise. That promise made up for your faults. And the promise I gave you made up for mine. Two imperfect people got married and it was the promise that made the marriage. And when our children were growing up, it wasn't a house that protected them; and it wasn't our love that protected them—it was that promise.

I wrote this book because I believe that the core social and personal challenge of our time is how to make loving, permanent marriage work for ourselves and our children. I fear that no social program, no educational achievement program, no job program, no anticrime program, and no amount of psychotherapy and Prozac will solve our society's problems unless we figure out how men and women can sustain permanent bonds that are good for them, their children, and their communities. Ours can't be the marriages of our parents and grandparents, because we live in an era that aspires to greater equality between men and women and to higher levels of emotional intimacy in marriage. But our communities are no less dependent on our success in forging bonds of love and cooperation in the home.

I wrote this book because I think that while our contemporary culture celebrates the consumer pleasures of getting married, it undermines our prospects for a permanent marriage. In a "me-first" world, marriage is a "we-first" contradiction.

I wrote this book because, even if we have an unbending commitment to our mates, most of us are blind to how we lose our marriages by slow erosion if we do not keep replenishing the soil. Modern marriages require more mindfulness than marriages of the past, because we expect more of marriage, but we have not yet woken up to that fact. We tend to focus on everything else but our marriage as the years go by. Success in marriage today requires two ingredients that no previous generation has ever had to put together: powerful commitment combined with an intentional focus on maintaining and growing one's marriage. Commitment without intentionality leads to stable but stale marriages. Intentionality without commitment leads to lively marriages that cannot endure bad weather.

I wrote this book because I think that friends and even professionals, such as psychotherapists, sometimes do more harm than good for our marriages, especially when we bring our complaints to them. I want people to be better able to find support for their marriages and to resist well-intentioned undermining from other people in their lives. A colleague told me that when she complains to her friends about her husband, their immediate response is often "Why are you still there?" She is completely committed to her marriage and is puzzled and troubled by her friends' well-intentioned but sabotaging comments.

I wrote this book to point out how we maintain too much privacy about our marriages and instead show how we can build supportive communities. A big part of my job as a marriage and family therapist is to show couples how widely shared their problems are. Think about how often most of us discuss the challenges, strategies, and joys of parenting, but how little we share the challenges, strategies, and joys of marriage. Solitary marriages are at-risk marriages in today's world. At our weddings, we take our citizenship papers in marriage as a publicly recognized social bond, but we have not learned how to practice this citizenship by taking responsibility for the welfare of all of our marriages.

This book differs from many other books on marriage because it does not deal extensively with communication skills, conflict management skills, and sexual relations. I wanted to write a book about matters that have not been emphasized as strongly in other books, in particular the themes of commitment, rituals of intentional marriage, and connections to community.

Updates to this book were based on research and cultural change over the past decade and my recent work with many couples on the brink of divorce. When I tell the stories of married couples in this book, I have disguised their identities. Some descriptions represent composite stories.

My thanks to Kitty Moore, my editor at The Guilford Press, who dreamed up the idea for this book with me, encouraged me to say what I wanted to say, gave me wise feedback on the first edition, encouraged me to write a second edition, and went several extra miles to make sure I was saying what I wanted to say. I am grateful to the many hundreds of couples who have trusted me with their stories, their strategies, and their pains over the past thirty-five years of my work as a marriage and family therapist. Although the stories I tell in this book reflect what they have taught me, I have disguised their identities and sometimes combined the experiences of different couples.

For a man of many words, I don't know how to express the fullness of my debt to my wife, Leah. No course, no professional training or experience, no workshop, no book—and none of these combined—has taught me as much about marriage as Leah has. She is a presence on every page.

While writing this book, I have thought of myself as in a relationship with you as a reader. I even noticed that I shared more personal stories in the second half of the book, after we had spent more "time" together. I would love to hear from you if you want to share your stories, to reflect on what reading this book has meant to you, or to tell me how you are taking action for your own marriage or the marriages in your community. You can contact me at *www. takebackyourmarriage.com.*

1 Take Back Your Marriage

Not far from my office in St. Paul, Minnesota, is the farthest point north on the Mississippi River where the big ships can navigate the river. Have you ever stood close to the edge of a river like the Mississippi? In most places the current is silent but formidable in strength. Everything on the water moves steadily south—or sometimes east or west for a while—but ultimately south toward New Orleans. Everything that is not powered by wind, gasoline, or human muscle.

Ever since I moved to Minnesota, I have thought that getting married is like launching a canoe into the Mississippi at St. Paul. If you don't paddle, you go south. No matter how much you love each other, no matter how full of hope and promise and good intentions, if you stay on the Mississippi without a good deal of paddling—occasional paddling is not enough—you end up in New Orleans. Which is a problem if you wanted to stay north.

At first, you are so captured by the joy of being married, so embraced by the good will of family and friends, that you hardly notice that you are passing Wabasha, Minnesota, on your slow drift south. After all, you are still in Minnesota. Next comes Dubuque, Iowa, but you are still in the upper Midwest. By the time you hit St. Louis, you know your marriage is not quite what you had hoped it would be, but it's still good and satisfying—just not as soaring and special as you had expected, given the great launching up north. If you can hold it together at St. Louis, that would be fine. But your muscles are out of shape now from too much sitting and too little paddling. (Recreational paddling is not enough to stay in one spot for long on the Mississippi; you've got to work at it.)

With two of you in the canoe, chances are that one of you becomes concerned about your marital drift well before St. Louis. One of you may comment about fewer long talks and about how little "quality time" you spend together now that your first child is in your life. Or one of you may complain about having sex less often and less passionately. For some couples, these complaints are a call to start paddling more vigorously. For other couples, the complaints lead to unpleasant arguments that lead to greater distance. But even when we are inspired to try harder, the extra work on our marriage tends to be short lived—sustained for days or weeks at best—and then we resume our slow drift south.

The problem is not lack of love or good intentions. The problem is that we don't understand the river currents, we don't have the mind-set to resist them, and we don't have a strategy for getting back north. In other words, we don't grasp what we are up against in contemporary marriage, so we don't have a master plan to take back our marriage when we start losing it. The result is that nearly all of us lose some parts of our marriage to the river current. If any of this fits you and your marriage, you are quite normal. The thing is, normal these days means you have to take back your marriage and head north time and again.

Why Our Marriages Drift

The natural drift of contemporary married life, in our busy, distracted, individualistic, cell phone–obsessed, consumer-driven, media-saturated, and work-oriented world, is toward less spark, less connection, less intimacy, and less focus on the couple relationship. Add in the demands of child-sensitive parenting, and you have a pretty good picture of why many marriages decline over time.

Is there a basis for these claims beyond my own opinion? Fortunately, marriage has been a well-researched topic in the social sciences. We know that about two-thirds of married couples begin a decline in their marital happiness after the birth of their first child. Like the Mississippi River current, the pulls on the relationship are steady and unrelenting during the childrearing years and beyond.

The good news is that recent research I've done with my colleague Jared Anderson has shown that about one in five couples start out well and go through no decline in their marital happiness over the years, and another forty-five percent have some decline and then bounce back.

You can take one of the best measures of marital happiness and see how you compare to national averages. (Note that this and several other practical tools from the book are available for downloading and printing at *www.guilford.com/p/doherty*.)

RATE YOUR MARITAL HAPPINESS: THE MARITAL HAPPINESS SCALE

I am now going to mention some different aspects of married life. For each one, I would like you to tell me whether you are very happy, pretty happy, or not too happy with this aspect of your marriage. If you are very happy, assign a number 3. If you are pretty happy, the number 2, and if not too happy, the number 1.

1. How happy are you with the amount of understanding you receive from your spouse?
2. How happy are you with the amount of love and affection you receive?
3. How happy are you with the extent to which you and your spouse agree about things?
4. How happy are you with your sexual relationship?
5. How happy are you with your spouse as someone who takes care of things around the house?
6. How happy are you with your spouse as someone to do things with?
7. How happy are you with your spouse's faithfulness to you?
8. Taking all things together, how would you describe your marriage?
9. Compared to other marriages you know about, do you think your marriage is better than most, about the same as most, or not as good as most?
10. Comparing your marriage to three years ago, is your marriage getting better (3), staying the same (2), or getting worse (1)?

For the last question, the response categories are a little different, but you still give yourself a 1, 2, or 3.

11. Would you say the feelings of love you have for your spouse are extremely strong (3), very strong (3), pretty strong (2), not too strong (1), or not strong at all (1)?

Now add up your total score. It can range from 11 to 33. Here is where your score fits with national norms for married people. The average marital happiness score is 29. The lowest twenty-fifth percentile is 27, which means that if your score was 27 or less, you are less happy with your marriage than 75 percent of married people. If your score was 32 or higher, you are more happily married than 75 percent of married people. Researchers have long noted that most people rate their marriages as happy, despite the nation's high divorce rate, perhaps because it's hard to admit dissatisfaction either to the researcher or to oneself. For that reason, a lower than average score is often a more reliable indicator of the state of someone's marriage. That is, you can accept at face value someone who indicates he or she is not so happy, but you have to assume that some people who score above average in happiness are doing a bit of wishful thinking.

From the Marital Instability over the Life Course Study conducted by Alan Booth and Paul Amato. This scale is in the public domain.

The upbeat research I just mentioned had one big limitation: it only measured couples who stayed together. What about couples whose boats don't just drift but crash on the rocks, the divorce casualties of marriage? One in four of all currently married couples are likely to divorce, and the projections for newly marrying couples is still in the forty to fifty percent range, the highest of any society in human history. The biggest risk for divorce is in the early years of marriage, with half of those who ever divorce doing so within the first six to seven years. (The recently reported increase in late-life divorces is a product of the high-divorcing baby boomers reaching older ages rather than a new risk in the later years of marriage.) The divorce rate for second marriages is even higher. With such large numbers of couples divorcing, and with many others drifting toward less satisfaction over the years, we clearly have a problem.

Later on, we will look in detail at the forces that drive even good marriages south. Here I want to highlight a few everyday factors, followed by a larger cultural one.

• We are too busy for our marriages. Between work, raising children, and managing daily life, many of us don't think we have enough time to make our marriage relationship a high priority in daily life.

• We get too used to our mate. In marriage, familiarity breeds not contempt, but taking each other for granted. All relationships lose some degree of newness and freshness over time if we don't work to put these ingredients back. Psychologists call it "habituation," a universal threat to intimate relationships. We stop dating, especially after we have children. Special alone times brought us together, but many of us stop arranging them after we become parents.

• We don't know other couples' strategies for maintaining vibrant marriages. In a culture of privacy about marriage, we don't share our struggles and successes with other couples. We drift pretty much in parallel formation, and when we do share, we tend to complain, and so do they.

• Differences between spouses in their "work orientation" toward marriage get resolved in the direction of less work. Our gender training as men and women prepares us differently for maintaining our marriages. At the risk of overgeneralizing, men tend to see close relationships as needing lower maintenance and work than women do. (Look at the difference in this regard between men's friendships and women's friendships.) Many wives, after a period of trying unilaterally to make the marriage a "high work" relationship, settle for their husband's standard. I don't want to overstate this gender difference, though, because often both spouses forget how to nurture their relationship over the long haul. And the current is too strong for that level of effort.

• Not only does the television absorb much of the rest of our attention during the day and evening, but many couples have a television in their bedrooms, thereby drawing eyes and ears away from each other at the only time of the day when they may have privacy.

• Then there is the rise of cells phones and social media which have transformed family communication since the first edition of this book. We now carry our computers in our hands. Some commentators claim that each of us has immediate access to more people and more information than presidents of the United States did a generation ago. The ultimate consequences for our marriages remain indeterminate, but it is clear that there are major threats. An obvious one is the development of online affairs, which therapists report are increasingly common issues in their offices. More generally, we can be so preoccupied with responding to our cell phones and engaging in online communication that we neglect our intimate relationships. We can have hundreds of Facebook friends and share things with them that we fail to mention to our spouse. Scholar Sherry Turkle argues from her research that technology offers the illusion of communication without any emotional risk, and the illusion of intimacy without the demands of intimacy. I'll return to this issue a number of times in this book.

Marriage and the Consumer Culture

The chief unrecognized enemy of marriage in today's world is the consumer culture of marketplace values, which has crept unnoticed into the family. In my book *Take Back Your Kids: Confident Parenting in Turbulent Times,* I argued that today's children are increasingly being raised as consumers of parental services, with parents seeing themselves as parental service providers to entitled children. Lost is the idea of children having responsibilities as citizens of families and communities. Well-intentioned parents anxiously provide their children every possible opportunity lest they fall behind in the competition to become successful adults. Parenting becomes product development.

The consumer culture has invaded marriage along with parenting, and it rides with us in the boat as we head south. The consumer attitude toward marriage is all around us and affects all of us, like global warming and air pollution. We can detect it most readily when we are bothered by something in our mate or our marriage and hear ourselves thinking or saying things like, "What am I getting out of this marriage, anyway?" Or "I deserve better!" or "What's in this for me?" Not that these thoughts are altogether inappropriate; if your spouse is having an affair or hitting you, then focusing on self-interest is quite appropriate. But when your mate is not the lover you had hoped for, or nags you more than you want, or is not emotionally expressive enough for you, then consumer thinking suggests that you have not cut the best possible deal in marrying this person. Then you start to do cost–benefit analysis: What am I getting from this relationship in terms of what I am putting into it?

I knew a couple who counted each time the other was out of town and owed an additional period of solo child care. Although they said they were trying to be fair to each other, I believe they were continually tallying what each was giving and receiving from the marriage. Later on, the husband left for another woman.

Not surprisingly, the pursuit of a good deal in an ongoing marriage makes it less likely that the marriage will be rewarding. Researcher Paul Amato has shown that focusing on "how is this going for me?" leads to less satisfaction with the marriage in the future than an attitude that is focused on commitment to the relationship. In my observation, when a husband keeps telling himself that he is entitled to better sex than he is getting in his marriage (a consumer attitude), he will continue to have an unsatisfying sexual relationship with his wife. She will not respond emotionally and erotically to his sense of entitlement. Spouses are supposed to be lovers, not providers of sexual and other marital services.

I recall the movie *Lovers and Other Strangers,* in which Bea Arthur, playing the mother of an adult son who has announced that he is getting a divorce because he is not happy in his marriage, delivers this great line: "Don't look for happiness, Richie, it will only make you miserable."

Perhaps you think I am exaggerating when I say that the consumer marketplace culture has invaded how we think about marriage. Advertisers know a cultural trend when they see one and are quick to use it to appeal to consumers. A magazine ad pictured a

new Honda Civic with the headline, "THE SAD THING IS, IT'LL PROBA-
BLY BE THE HEALTHIEST RELATIONSHIP OF YOUR ADULT LIFE." Honda
explains: *"You've tried the personals, blind dates, even one of those
online chat rooms. Why? The Civic Sedan is smart, fun, reliable and
good-looking. Not to mention, it's ready to commit, today."* Then, lest
the reader feel suddenly commitment-shy, the ad ends in the wink
of a headlight: *"Looking for a good time?"*

Apparently we must seek "healthy adult relationships" with
cars because, as an ad for Levi's jeans has recognized, marriage
can't be counted on anymore. In a lavish six-page spread we see
happy dating couples, with captions announcing how long they were
together before breaking up. The final page shows two female roommates, one consoling the other about a recent breakup. Just behind
the two roommates, on the kitchen wall, is an art poster with the
Spanish words *Mis padres se divorcian:* "My parents are divorced."
The caption underneath delivers the ad's take-home message: "At
least some things last forever—Levi's: they go on."

The message is that we can only count on what we buy, not on
what we share or the people to whom we commit ourselves. And the
only role that endures is that of consumer. Companies that want
our business will do whatever it takes to meet our needs, unlike
our spouses, who sometimes put their own needs, or the children's
needs, before ours. Levi's will be there for us, even if our parents
divorce and our lovers leave us. How comforting.

At the heart of today's consumer culture is the idea that our
purchases and our relationships should be therapeutic, good for us
psychologically. Marriage is (or used to be) our culture's most cherished venue for personal growth and fulfillment. But steadfastness
and self-sacrifice are not in this picture of therapeutic consumption.
When the marriage relationship becomes psychologically painful or
stunts our growth, there are plenty of therapists around to serve as
midwives for a divorce. And most baby boomers and their offspring
have an internalized therapist in our heads—the psychological voice
of the consumer culture—to encourage us to stop working so hard or
to get out of a marriage that is not meeting our current emotional
needs. In consumer marriage, the customer—you or me as individuals pursuing our just rewards—is always right.

In 2009 many watched with fascination the results of the infidelities of Tiger Woods. I was struck not just with what Tiger did to his marriage (chronic infidelity has always been with us), but with the message his father, Earl, had left him with. Not only did Earl Woods himself have trouble settling down and being faithful to one woman, he was also a perceptive observer of the culture. Here is what Karen Crouse of *The New York Times* wrote: "Woods's parenting role model was his father, Earl, who was committed to rearing him after having two sons and a daughter in a failed first marriage. . . . Perhaps Woods was destined to be like his father, only not in the way he had hoped. Over lunch on the veranda at the Masters one year, Earl Woods said, 'I've told Tiger that marriage is unnecessary in a mobile society like ours.'" This is more than a fetching celebrity anecdote. We know from research that children of divorce have a fifty percent increase in their odds of divorce, and that ambivalence about whether lifelong commitment is possible is a likely factor in that risk. Children of divorce aspire to lifelong marriage but are not as confident they can achieve it.

Intentional Marriage

I want to tell you a story of Ken and Judy, a couple I saw in therapy back when I was living in Oklahoma. They made a beautiful pair—tall, handsome, and graceful. They had met on the country-western dance floor, and they told me, with a touch of shyness, that they were really good dancers. So good that other people on the dance floor would sometimes make a circle and watch them dance. Ken and Judy had been married for three years. When I asked them when was the last time they had danced, they replied ruefully, "Three years ago." The ritual that brought them together—that helped to define them as a couple—was something they had abandoned. Dance floors, I guess, are for singles and for couples who are falling in love, not for married couples trying to sustain their love.

We fall in love through rituals of connection and intimacy—courtship rituals like romantic dinners, long talks, riding bicycles or going skiing, going for walks, exchanging gifts, talking every night on the telephone. We mostly do these rituals alone as a couple; when people are falling in love, their family and friends know to give them some space. We gladly fill our time through rituals of connection and intimacy. We develop a common language and a common experience bank. We go to dinner at our favorite spots, and we try to sit at our favorite tables. We go dancing at our favorite places. And we don't dance with everybody in the room; we dance mostly with the person we are falling in love with. And then we get married.

Why do we give up what made us so happy at an earlier phase in our relationship? Falling in love is the ultimate consumer fantasy, up there with a truly wonderful SUV or townhouse. Growing the new relationship and reaping personal rewards go hand in hand. When things go well, I give to you, you give to me, and we are wonderful as a couple. What's more, our passion is fueled by anxiety about whether the relationship will last. Romance, novelty, and fear of loss—the stuff of operas and love affairs.

A courtship like Ken and Judy's, when the feelings are right, is easy to prioritize in one's life. But it takes mindfulness and self-discipline to make the relationship a priority once we have made a permanent commitment and begun to live as a family. During courtship, and in the early months for couples who live together, the relationship is figural in our lives—front and center, if you will— and the rest of our lives are background. When we get married, and particularly after we have children, this reverses. Other things— the children, our work, our hobbies, even our religious involvement—become central or figural, and the marriage recedes to the background and only gets our attention when something is wrong. An intentional marriage, unlike an intentional courtship, is a high achievement because it requires the discipline to keep connecting when natural energies and passions ebb.

What do I mean by an intentional marriage? It's one in which the partners are conscious, deliberate, and planful about maintaining and building their commitment and connection over the years. They see themselves as active citizens of their marriage rather than as passive consumers of marital services. A lot goes into being intentional about marriage. I place special emphasis on three aspects: a rock-solid commitment to the marriage, a reservoir of marital rituals of connection and intimacy, and a supportive community. There are other ways to be intentional as well, such as developing good communication skills and constructive ways to argue and deal with conflict. In this era, if we are not intentional, we will become a consumer couple that has bought the boat and expects love and good intentions, and for the river to do the rest.

The only way to take back our marriages from their drift south is to keep paddling and have a joint navigational plan. Paddling means doing the everyday things to stay connected, to find time for each other, to go on dates, to make a big deal of anniversaries and special occasions, to work hard to reconnect after periods when we have been distracted from each other. Having a joint navigational plan means that you both are committed for keeps, with no exit strategy, and that you both take responsibility to monitor how the marriage is doing, when it needs midcourse corrections, and when it needs help in the form of marriage education or marital therapy. Intentional marriage is about everyday attention and long-range planning.

One of the ironies of contemporary family life is that many people who are good at intentional parenting are lousy at intentional marriage. We evolve good parent–child rituals over the years, but we lose our marital rituals. People can be quite gifted at rituals with the whole family—family dinners, camping trips, vacations—and quite dumbfounded about what they would do as a couple. Couples who courted through long, romantic dinners are sometimes nervous about dining alone because they are not sure what they would say to each other for an hour or more. So they make sure to invite other people along for company. When it comes to long-range planning, many of us are good at thinking about our children's future but lousy at thinking about how we will be a couple when our children are older. If we are honest, how many of us would give ourselves the same "letter grade" for effort in our marriage as for effort in our parenting? How many of us would die before putting our parenting on hold for weeks but end up putting our marriage on hold for years?

Frank and Sally are a good example of a couple who started out devoted to each other and then transferred this devotion to their children. Always active people who used to bike and camp together as a couple, they now are highly engaged in their children's sports, music, and other activities. They do as many of these activities together as possible, so it's not like they go in separate directions all the time. They have friends they do things with, including family camping events. But the spark of emotional intimacy has gradually faded from their marriage. They never go out on dates. They go to bed at different times because Frank likes to stay up later. Sex has become infrequent. They celebrate their anniversary by going out with another couple. They still love each other and are fully committed to their marriage and family life. And they have the seeds of good companionship and good will toward each other. But when they allow themselves to reflect on their early dreams for their marriage, they feel some sadness—a sadness quickly countered by the thought that this is how marriage is after you have children and a busy life.

I am not saying that Frank and Sally have chosen the wrong path in life; there are many ways to be married and few of us achieve all of our initial life goals. But a couple that does not have an intentional marriage place themselves at risk for the infiltration of consumer marriage. One day either Frank or Sally might start to think, "Is this all that life offers me? Am I really happy in this marriage? Could somebody give me more intimacy in my life?" I have seen too many people turn a critical eye on their spouse when they start feeling twinges of sadness about the marriage that might have been. After all, if they're not happy, as good consumers they must assume it's because their mate is a poor marital service provider or that the original "purchase" was a mistake. In that case, the only thing to do is to find a new canoe mate to start the journey all over again, leaving the wreckage of children's and adults' lives on the water. But the Mississippi will play no favorites with the next marriage either.

The main way to resist the forces that pull us apart—the natural drift of marriage over time and the insidious pull of the consumer culture—is to be a couple who carefully cultivates their commitment and ways to connect over the years. Simply stated, the intentional couple thinks about their relationship, plans for their relationship, and acts for their relationship, mostly in simple, everyday ways and occasionally in big, splashy ways.

Two Kinds of Marital Commitment

Commitment is the starter motor of a marriage. It not only launches us when we marry, but we crank it every day. We especially call on it when things are not going well. I want to talk about two kinds of commitment—a tentative one and a permanent one. In long-term follow-up studies of new married couples, psychologist Thomas Bradbury and his colleagues have shown that it makes a big difference whether people think of commitment as something like "I like this relationship and I want to stay in it," versus something like "I will do what it takes to make this relationship successful even when times are hard."

Janna and Sebastian are taking the more tentative approach to commitment that is increasingly popular among couples who live together—and even among those who get married. They are committed as long as they make each other happy, as long as they get along, as long as their individual life goals line up, as long as neither betrays the other's trust by having an affair, as long as they don't fight too much, as long as the sex is good, as long as the relationship meets their needs and helps them grow as people. I call this "commitment for now." The bottom line is to stay together, not as long as we both shall live, but as long as things are working out for me.

Every important cultural trend and every form of commitment that many couples embrace has something to teach us and that we should not lose sight of. "Commitment for now" stresses that commitment is a choice, not just a cultural mandate. It embraces the importance of spouses advocating for their needs and rights in the relationship. It emphasizes that people should not sit still while being taken advantage of by their spouses. It promotes self-advocacy in marriage for both women and men. But while this kind of commitment works well for courting or cohabiting couples who are exploring whether to make a permanent commitment, it lacks the staying power for the long haul of a marriage. It's a starter motor designed to be used for months or years but not decades, and for good weather conditions but not for bad ones.

The other kind of commitment is not tentative. I call it "commitment for the long haul." This is the long view of marriage in which you don't balance the ledgers every month to see whether you are getting an adequate return on your investment. You have signed citizenship papers in a new country, which is now your country, and you don't have a plan for how to expatriate if the nation's economy goes sour or the political winds blow in directions you don't like. You are here to stay.

Long-haul commitment combines elements of traditional religious and moral commitment with newer elements that recognize that marriage must be an intentional process of shared maintenance and renewal. This modern form of permanent commitment puts together the traditional ideal of an unbreakable marital covenant with the modern notions of gender equality, psychological intimacy, and focused work on growing a relationship. Also, let me be clear that it is possible for a spouse to lose a just claim on the commitment of the partner by a consistent pattern of misconduct and abuse of the marital vows. There are tragic exceptions when permanent commitment must be withdrawn. But that does not deter us from making the initial commitment anyway. That's what makes it so scary, and the potential rewards so extraordinary.

Community-Based Marriage versus Solitary Marriage

Consumer marriage is not only passive. It is also solitary, as opposed to being rooted in a community. As consumers in the marketplace, we make individual decisions to purchase or not purchase a product or service. It may be for our family, but it's still a private, personal matter. We don't buy a new television set for the neighborhood. The consumer culture consists of lots of individuals doing what they think is best for themselves, guided by mass advertising. Even when we resist the force of individualism by seeing ourselves as a loving, committed couple, most of us still go through married life without a lot of give and take with a community of people concerned about the welfare of our marriage. As I said before, we talk about almost everything else in our lives—our kids, parents, jobs, health—but relatively little about our marriages. We don't know what goes on inside other people's marriages, and we are reluctant to ask. When we do talk, it's apt to be in the form of complaints.

I like to ask clergy to compare the number of people in their congregation whom they can freely ask about their health, their personal stress level, or worries about their jobs or kids with the number whom they can ask about how their marriages are doing. With some embarrassment, most clergy tell me that the second number is very low indeed in comparison to the first. After the wedding, our marriages tend to be invisible in our faith communities, unless we get to the brink of divorce.

For the most part, we know our friends' birthdays better than their wedding anniversaries, and we celebrate the birthdays more. How many times have you been shocked to learn that a friend's or family member's marriage is on the rocks, when you would have certainly known about a serious health problem? Marriage is too important, and too difficult, to do without a supportive community. But we are babes at learning how to create community for our marriages.

Taking Back Our Marriages

What I can offer you is a vision of resistance, a vision of renewal, and some tools for crafting an intentional marriage for your journey. The vision of resistance is that we band together, in our marriages and our communities, to resist the social forces and cultural currents that pull us apart faster than our love and good intentions can bring us back together again. This is a culture war worth fighting, for the stakes are high. We must name these forces that undermine marriage, from the small forces such as boredom to the big ones such as the throwaway consumer culture and the despair in some of our communities that a good marriage is even possible.

We must become adept at recognizing the drift of our marriages and the insinuating influence of marketplace values, and we must learn ways to counteract them. Like all forms of human resistance, this struggle is best undertaken not just by individuals in their personal lives—taking back our marriages one couple at a time—but also by all of us together in community. You no doubt have discovered your own ways to resist these forces and keep your marriage alive. Perhaps you go out on dates as a couple, or celebrate your anniversary in a meaningful way. Perhaps you counteract the entitled, me-first thoughts that impede partnership, or work to keep your sexual relationship alive even when you are tired a lot of the time. As you read this book, I hope you will recognize and celebrate how you already resist the forces that threaten all of our marriages, that you will discover new ways to resist as a couple, and that you will find ways to band together with other couples in the struggle.

A vision of renewal goes hand in hand with resistance. We can be architects of our own marriages, our own shipbuilders, if you will. If we construct our own oars, we are more apt to use them because they fit us. Aside from your individual efforts for your own marriage, I invite you to think of yourself as a supporter of marriage as social institution and central human bond. In other words, I invite you to care about the health of marriage in our culture, just as you care about the strength of our schools and the viability of our health care system. It may seem like a strange suggestion in a book that focuses on the personal side of the marital relationship, but I invite you to try it on for size.

In this book we will explore together three paths to marital renewal, all of which combined constitute what I think of as an intentional marriage in today's world:

- Being mindful and focused on your relationship rather than drifting.
- Being committed for the long haul rather than committed "as long as."
- Being communal rather than solitary.

I hope to teach you the skills of having an intentional marriage in a world that pulls us apart. In addition to helping you see the big picture of today's marriages and what research has to offer, I have lots of practical ideas to pass on to you, some I've learned with my wife in our marriage, and others I've learned from couples I've known and worked with. An example is how to construct a "talk ritual" for fifteen minutes per day, just for you and your mate. This is a high accomplishment for a married couple with growing children and something that must be carefully constructed or it won't last a week. Marriage requires a good deal of know-how, some of which you already have and some of which I can help you learn.

Binding and Clinging

In his wonderful play *Joe Turner's Come and Gone,* the playwright August Wilson has a character who is a healer in an early twentieth-century African American community in Pittsburgh. One day the healer is bragging that he can help any couple bind their relationship. A friend challenges him about whether he can help even those who are not meant to be together. The healer clarifies: "I'm a Binder of What Clings. You got to find out if they cling first." And then he offers these words that become the refrain of the play: "You can't bind what don't cling." You can't bind what don't cling. Without the glue of commitment, nothing else binds us together for the long and winding road of marriage. This glue is mostly a decision, a choice to be together and stay together through better and worse.

I once worked with a very distressed couple whose perseverance was a marvel to me. Most couples would have given up long ago. It was one of those rare times where I was ready to give up before they were. It just seemed so hopeless. One time, I said, "I've run out of ideas. I've got nothing more. But I'll go around the track again with you if you want." And they said, "Yeah, we want to stay with it." And they eventually found each other again. I asked them how they had endured these dark days. They said that they had clung to their Friday Shabbat meal, their religious ritual in their Jewish tradition—even if they were not speaking to each other. No matter how bad things were, whether they were not sleeping together or not speaking together, they never missed this ritual, which gave them hope. The hope sprang from their ability to work together to keep their family's religious tradition intact. You can't bind what don't cling.

Only when we hold each other tight through adversity and honestly face up to the distance we have come from our hopes and ideals for our marriage, can we unleash our capacity for renewal. We are then free to exercise our skills in the crafts of maintaining our canoe, paddling together, and navigating the big river to where we want to go instead of where it wants to take us.

2 Resisting Consumer Marriage

I want to tell you about Cheryl, who had been married for seventeen years and had two teenage daughters. About a year ago, she began an affair with a man she knew professionally. Her job took her out of town about once a month, when she and her lover got together for great sex and conversation. Right now, her lover, recently divorced from his wife, was pressing Cheryl for a commitment to leave her husband and be with him.

I asked about her marriage. She said that her husband was a very good man—"kind and loving and supportive" were her words—but that the marriage lacked passion for her. She had felt emotionally empty for a number of years. They were doing a good job raising their children, she thought. They rarely argued. Their sexual relationship had been "blah" for many years—infrequent and unexciting. Her husband had supported her career decisions, although they did not share many outside interests. In fact, he was so supportive and constructive that she was confident that he would not abandon her or be mean-spirited if she told him about the affair. Although being hurt terribly, he would work to make things better, she said. But Cheryl told herself and me that she deserved more out of life and marriage than she felt she could get from her husband. It was fear of hurting her children that was most stopping her from leaving. They would be devastated, she thought, and their lives turned upside down, especially if she was the one to move out and away to the community where her lover lived.

Cheryl was facing what she called a "churning dilemma." She

didn't "fall" into the affair, she noted; she had clearly decided to pursue something she felt she needed and deserved in her life. Her lover gave her more than her husband; she felt far better when she was with him. Their conversations were deeper and their sex more thrilling. After years of passively accepting a loving but "blah" marriage, she felt that she had come alive after being kissed by a man who had been her friend but soon became her lover.

I don't want to portray Cheryl as hopelessly self-centered; in fact, she was very concerned about the effects of her actions on her family. Cheryl struck me as a good and sensitive person caught between her conscience and her desires for more in her life. But she spoke about her personal desires as if they were constitutional rights, such as freedom of speech, and her emotional needs as if they were biological facts, such as needing vitamin C to avoid scurvy. Our culture teaches us that we are all entitled to an exciting marriage and great sex life; if we don't get both, we are apt to feel deprived. What used to be seen as human weakness of the flesh has become a personal entitlement.

Social historians have shown how psychological individualism has been growing in our nation for more than a century. Its current form is what I call the consumer attitude, a combination of the human potential movement of the 1970s (with its focus on personal growth) and the market values that came to dominate starting in the 1980s (with their focus on personal entitlement and cutting your losses and moving on if you are not satisfied).

Although the consumer attitude lurks inside nearly every married person who lives in our culture, it often does not become apparent until we come face to face with our disappointments about our marriage and our mate. That's when we start to ask ourselves, "Is this marriage meeting my needs?" and "Am I getting enough back for what I am putting into this marriage?" In Cheryl's case, she had told herself for years that she was staying in the marriage only for the sake of the children. She had "settled" for a second-class marriage in a world that tells us not to settle for second best, because a better product or service is beckoning. Hence she was vulnerable to enticements of a new relationship that looked like it could make her truly happy.

I invite you to train your ear to the sound of consumer marriage in the world around you and in your own head. The sound is easiest to detect in the media, culture, and other people's marriages, like Cheryl's. So we will start outside. And then we will listen inside our own marriages—yours and mine.

Consumer Marriage in the Media and Culture

We talked before about how marketers for Honda and Levi's have picked up the consumer marriage theme. Here are some other media and cultural snippets: A *New York Times* journalist reports hearing a guest at a wedding reception, presumably a relative of the groom, say about the bride: "She will make a nice first wife for Jason." One national family expert endorses what she terms "starter marriages"—marriages that are good learning experiences but not likely to endure. Does this make you think of a "starter house" that you expect to sell once you can afford something better? A California futurologist uses the term "ice-breaker" marriage to mean the same thing. In a *Time* magazine piece on predicting the future of male–female relationships, feminist social critic Barbara Ehrenreich trumpets "renewable marriages," which "get re-evaluated every five to seven years, after which they can be revised, recelebrated, or dissolved with no, or at least fewer, hard feelings." These critics of marriage make a good point in stressing the importance of renewing marital commitment time and again, but their skepticism about permanent commitment ironically makes it less likely that couples will last long enough to renew their marriages again and again.

What we used to think of as our first love—our first intense dating relationship when we were immature and not ready for a commitment—has now become our first marriage. And what we used to think of as a contract with a bank—for a five-year renewable mortgage—has become the metaphor for our marriages.

Listen also for our contemporary humor about marriage. A joke I heard when visiting the Boston area goes this way: "When choosing a husband, ask yourself if this is the man you want your children to visit every other weekend." A character in a recent movie says that men should be like toilet paper: soft, strong, and disposable. A woman in a *New Yorker* cartoon tells her friend, "He's very well off. He's got all the quantities I admire."

Having a spouse or leaving a spouse increasingly sounds like a consumer purchase or sale decision. Interviewed about her life, a never-married woman with two small children tells *The New York Times*, "I'm a single mother. It's just me. At a certain age I realized I didn't want to be a wife. Now I can see why some women have husbands. It's kind of a convenience." An expert on extramarital affairs, when asked by *Psychology Today* whether she ever counsels people directly to leave a relationship, replies in the language of the marketplace: "Leaving a bad marriage without trying to repair it first is like buying high and selling low. Better to see how good you can make it, then look at it and ask: Is this good enough?" Of course there is wisdom in this advice, but I also find it chilling. The same advice would apply to a new car that needs repairs.

Beyond listening to contemporary discourse, just look at contemporary behavior. A Philadelphia couple who desired a more expensive wedding than they could afford got twenty-four companies to sponsor the wedding in exchange for having their company names appear six times on everything from the invitations to the thank-you notes. At the other end of the marriage journey, lawyers pay for billboards advertising cheap, quick divorces.

Here's one more example of the commercialization of marital commitment. Some years ago Toyota had an advertisement in the form of a "prenuptial agreement," with the use of quasi-legal language and names of three attorneys at the top of the page. The text begins with the acknowledgment by the parties—the customer and the automobile—of their "decision to marry each other and to enter in this Agreement." The prenuptial goes on to discuss arrangements about "separate property" and "earned and unearned property." The legal formalities out of the way, the ad's punch line is "Let the romance begin with a Camry Solara." Before long, Toyota will come out with a new, improved model, and we will be grateful that the prenuptial will smooth the trade-in process with our current car. As I said, advertisers know social trends when they see them. Consumer marriage is now fully in vogue.

Al and Tipper Gore's divorce in 2010 was a cultural bellwether for the consumer culture of marriage. This couple had survived the near death of a child, Tipper's depression, and Al's cliff-hanger loss of the presidency. They wrote a book titled *Joined at the Heart*. They were the baby-boomer couple who could.

Listen to their public statement: they had come to a "mutual and mutually supportive decision that we have made together following a process of long and careful consideration." They left family friends and former spokespersons to fill in a story line that went like this in *The New York Times*: The Gores "had grown apart after decades," and especially "after Al moved onto a global stage while Tipper seemed to move in a more personal direction." One close friend added that "there's not a lot of drama behind this . . . they remain very close friends."

Is this little whimper all that a forty-year marriage with children and grandchildren is worth? Sports teams and their home cities show more grief and anger when teams leave for better stadiums and tax benefits. The breakups of authors and literary agents, political candidates and campaign managers, come with more public emotion. Without revealing details that the public has no right to know, would it be too much for the Gores to say something like "This is really hard and involves a lot of pain and regret." In truth, their divorce story line is a non-statement like the ones we hear from Hollywood couples who break up with nothing but civility and remain "best of friends."

More than anything else, what concerns me about the Gore divorce is the cultural message it reinforces: that marriages, like oil spills, drift in ways that we can't do much about, that people once mated for life get caught in different currents and wake up one morning to find themselves in different seas, too far apart to be life partners any more. This message fits the easy come–easy go consumer culture to perfection. But I do not accept this pseudo-sophisticated story line for modern marriage. I do not accept the baby-boom divorce mantra that "these things happen to the best of marriages; let's be civilized and not show how we feel about the end of a dream." When it comes to divorce, I'm with the poet Dylan Thomas when he wrote about death:

Do not go gentle into that good night.
Rage, rage against the dying of the light.

How Did We Get Here?

Let me put consumer marriage in a bigger context. According to Lizabeth Cohen in her masterful book *A Consumer Republic: The Politics of Mass Consumption in Post-War America,* the consumer culture began in the late nineteenth century with the development of mass-produced commodities and the subsequent advent of the advertising industry. Advertisers realized that the key to successful marketing was convincing potential customers that they couldn't do without the product. Sometimes this meant defining new problems, such as bad breath and hairy legs, that new products would fix. If a company's product was indistinguishable in quality from another's—say, with gasoline, soft drinks, or cigarettes—then advertisers learned to sell an image, a sense of belonging, of having made it, of being with it.

During the Great Depression in the 1930s, public officials were alarmed at the decline in consumer spending and called on good Americans to buy consumer goods in order to revive the economy. This was the first connection between citizenship and consumerism. During World War II the message was reversed: sacrifice, save, and don't expect to spend on consumer goods. The government needed to spend the available money. After the war the big fear of economists and government leaders was that Americans would not spend the higher wages they were earning. The government responded by subsidizing mortgages and encouraging the housing boom in the suburbs. Business responded with malls and other new shopping opportunities away from the core cities. What Cohen calls "The Consumer Republic" was born, with an ever-growing hold of the mind-set on American life. Richard Nixon was credited with soundly defeating Soviet Premier Nikita Khrushchev in the much-trumpeted "kitchen debate" in 1959 by showcasing the superior kitchen appliances of American housewives.

Over the subsequent forty years, the consumer culture continued to morph. First was the advent of consumer niche markets: not mass-produced products for everyone, but specific markets for youth, women, men, parents, singles, and minority groups. We are now in an era of "identity consumption"—asserting one's unique identity by the goods and services we buy. You can see wedding trends following the same trajectory, from a standard wedding to niche weddings and now to weddings where couples want to "brand" their wedding with their unique personalities and tastes. As my daughter, Elizabeth Doherty Thomas, and I wrote in our book *Take Back Your Wedding,* American brides and grooms have absorbed the cultural message that their wedding is all about them, and little about their families and communities. I have no problem with couples deciding on a small, private wedding, but when they invite their social world to celebrate with them, the wedding should take these people into account. Contemporary weddings combine the identity consumer culture with the entitled celebrity culture—quite a way to launch a marriage that will succeed only if these two cultures are resisted.

Cohen argues that consumer culture is now the dominant force in American life. At the economic level, consumer spending is two-thirds of our economy. At the cultural level, consumerism is the dominant metaphor in nearly all areas, including education, medicine, religion, and politics. Why would we not expect it to invade marriage and family life?

Lest I seem to be against markets and against consumption, let me reassure you. From my perspective, there is no viable alternative to free-market democratic systems, and no feasible way to eliminate advertising without wreaking havoc on the economy, throwing millions of people out of work, and creating unworkable government bureaucracies. Consumer spending is the primary fuel of a free-market economy, and consumer spending relies on advertising to potential customers. The marketplace is necessary and here to stay, as is the consumer orientation it supports.

My concern is less with consumer culture in the marketplace than with what it is teaching us about our family relationships. Consumer culture tells us that we never have enough of anything we want, that the new is always better than the old—unless something old becomes trendy again. It teaches us not to be loyal to anything or anyone that does not continue to meet our needs at the right price. Customers are inherently disloyal. I want to support American workers, but have always bought Japanese cars because I have seen them as superior to American cars for the same price. I eat Cheerios for breakfast every day, but if the price gets too much higher than Special K, my second choice, I will abandon Cheerios. Or if General Mills changes the recipe, I might jump ship. I owe nothing to those who sell to me except my money, which I can stop giving at any time.

We Americans are also less apt to stay put now than in the past; we move where there are jobs and where we can afford to live. I know families who have chosen to stay in declining neighborhoods because they are involved in their community and because they don't want to encourage more middle-class flight from the inner city, but mostly we live where we can meet our personal and family needs. Studies of religious participation show that we are less loyal to particular religious denominations, churches, and other faith communities; we shop for the best religious experience.

Our children have picked up this consumer attitude, as I pointed out in *Take Back Your Kids*. When reminded by his father to do his chore of mowing the lawn, a fifteen-year-old boy replied, "It's not my lawn." When an eleven-year-old boy failed to thank his father for a Hanukkah gift, his mother admonished him for not saying thank you. The boy's response: "Why should I? I don't like it." These were "good kids," not problem kids, in good families with loving parents, but influenced by the individualistic consumer culture. A sixteen-year-old girl was incredulous that anyone would expect to have a common family dinner on a regular basis. With complete innocence, she asked a National Public Radio reporter, "How can we be expected to eat together if we are not all hungry at the same time?" Children have come to see themselves, under our tutelage and that of the marketplace, only as consumers of parental and community services and not as citizens with responsibilities to families and communities.

Even in parents' attitudes toward their children, I see the creeping language of the me-first consumer culture. In the past decade I have begun to hear parents of teenagers say things like, "What am

I getting out of being a parent to this kid?" and "When do I start to get something in return?" These parents love their children but are stressed by the job of parenting. It was when I began to hear this kind of cost–benefit consumer language from well-intentioned parents that I decided to start speaking out. It's insidious, and it leads good people to do bad things in their families and communities. An upper-middle-class father with plenty of resources tells his wife that he cannot take the stress of their sixteen-year-old daughter's behavior problems. "She is trying to tear us apart," he declares, and tells his wife that either their daughter leaves or he leaves. The daughter gets the message and moves out, returning later pregnant and on drugs. In the late 1960s, shelters were set up for teens who ran away from what they thought were overcontrolling parents. In Minneapolis, the oldest such shelter now has a bigger category of youth than "runaways." The majority now fits the category of "throwaway youth" whose parents have said "enough." I should point out that the behavior of most of these youth is not worse than in previous generations. What has changed is parents' commitment to accept long periods where their "costs" outweigh their "benefits" from the difficult job of parenting. I find it a frightening trend.

It is not surprising that in this new consumer world, we are less loyal to our mates, to our marriages. And when a marriage breaks up, it is not surprising that one of the parents exits from the children's lives to create a new life and a new family. I know a number of fathers who invest emotionally and financially in the children of their new wife but let go of their obligations to their own children who stay with their previous wife. These men have cut their losses and moved on. And it's not just fathers. One woman told me that her mother's parting words, upon leaving the family, were that she needed to pursue her dreams in life.

That was a common exit line in the 1970s, and the consumer version of it continues to this day. Elaine, a woman who suddenly left her empty but low-conflict marriage, decided to live with a friend who did not have space for her teenage daughter, whom she left with her stepfather, feeling rejected and abandoned. When asked for an explanation, Elaine explained that she had decided she needed to start making her own needs a higher priority. She had felt "stuck" and decided one weekend to act, because life is short. In a dramatic family therapy session in which Elaine gave this explanation for her actions, Elaine's stepdaughter (her husband's child who only visited on weekends) expressed admiration for this woman who would make a decision to "go for it" to have a better life. (I felt like I was listening to a beer commercial about "going for the gusto" because "we only go around once in life.") Elaine's own daughter turned to her stepsister and quietly uttered the most powerful refutation I have ever heard in a therapy session: "But she's got kids." Elaine's jaw dropped. Shortly after this confrontation, she moved to her own apartment and took her daughter in. But a lot of damage had been done. The good news is that Elaine over time recovered her sense of responsibility and became a real mother to her daughter. The marriage did not survive, however.

It is not new to our species that people abandon their responsibilities. We are all weak at times, and all tempted. What's new is the cultural support for a me-first approach to life, an invisible but powerful chemical in the air we breathe.

The sociologist Arlie Hochschild observed that in the new American lifestyle, rootlessness occurs on a global scale. "We move not only from one job to another, but from one spouse—and sometimes one set of children—to the next. We are changing from a society that values employment and marriage to one that values employability and marriageability." You see, it is your ability to love, not the people you love, that counts as a permanent asset in the consumer culture of relationships. A particular relationship may not continue to satisfy your needs, but you will be happy in life if you have the skills to attract and land a new lover. This approach has merit when seeking a lifelong mate (after all, most love relationships break up before marriage), but when it carries over into marriage itself, we keep our romantic resumes up to date in case this marriage does not work out. This tentativeness then makes the marriage less likely to work out.

What happens when we approach marriage and family life as entrepreneurs? When the initial glow fades and the tough times come, we are prepared to cut our losses, to take what we want from our old marriages in order to forge new, more perfect unions until they also must be dissolved. Where does it end? Even worse than the results of business layoffs, there are few soft landings after marital downsizing.

During the go-go economic years of the 1980s and 1990s, when market economies triumphed over socialist economies all over the world, the consumer culture captured the hearts—and marriages—of Americans in new ways. (As I said before, the consumer ethic of relationships was the culmination of the spirit of individualism that has been growing gradually for more than a century.) Mid-twentieth-century marriage, which featured high expectations for personal satisfaction, mutated into consumer marriage, with the same high psychological expectations but now spiced with a sense of entitlement and impermanence. The chief value of consumer marriage is making sure that one's needs are being met and that one's options are always open.

In practice, most couples embrace a variety of values for their marriage, including the values of responsibility and commitment. It's not that we suddenly have become selfish louts. But these values are always in danger of being trumped by the consumer values of personal gain, low cost, entitlement, and hedging one's bets. In consumer culture, the exit door is always accessible. Commitments last as long as the other person is meeting our needs. We still believe in commitment, but powerful voices coming from inside and outside tell us that we are suckers if we settle for less than we think we need and deserve in our marriage.

Consumer Marriage and Unnecessary Divorce

Reasons people give for getting a divorce reveal how they think about marital commitment. I have seen a shift over nearly thirty-five years of practice as a marriage and family therapist, a shift supported by research studies. I don't mean to say that most people are not experiencing real emotional pain at the time they decide to end their marriages. It's just that the reasons they give are far different from the hard, nasty problems that propelled spouses in

previous generations to divorce: abuse, abandonment, chronic alcoholism, infidelity—what I call the "hard reasons" for divorce. When
one's spouse will not change these behaviors, divorce may be necessary. My concern is with the "soft reasons" that are related to the
consumer culture of marriage.

Nowadays many people explain their reasons for divorce in the
form of disappointment in what they are getting from their marriage, rather than in the form of an unconscionable breakdown of
marital responsibilities. Here are phrases that I hear in my therapy
practice and in my personal life.

"The relationship wasn't working for me anymore."
"Our needs were just too different."
"I wasn't happy."
"We just grew apart."
"I grew and he didn't."
"She has changed too much."
"I deserve more."
"We are not the same people we were when we got married."
"After the children left home, there was nothing left."
"The relationship became stale."
"My husband was a nice guy, but boring."
"We had no real intimacy. What kind of role model is that for
    the kids?"

I used to take many of these as valid reasons to end a marriage.
If the marriage is not meeting your needs, especially if you have
tried hard to change it, then it is reasonable to leave. But as my
career moved on and I saw more of the ongoing pain of divorce for
adults and children, and as I saw people returning to therapy in the
second marriages with similar complaints, I grew more doubtful. As
I describe more fully in Chapter 7, you can work your way out of a
reasonably good marriage by focusing on what you are not getting
out of it and turning negative toward your mate, who will in turn
give you even less and thereby help justify your leaving.

I think of a husband who could not accept the fact that his wife
had gone back to graduate school and become a religious liberal

instead of a religious conservative. He felt personally affronted by her changes and hounded her out of the marriage. She was an emotional wreck by the time she decided to divorce, and then he acted as if the divorce was her doing. Theirs had been an okay marriage, not a wonderful one, and good for their children. I used to explain this kind of divorce in neutral terms, such as "they grew in different directions," or "she outgrew him," or "he was too rigid for her." But nowadays I see the husband as responsible for creating an unnecessary divorce by his refusal to deal with his disappointment in his wife's changes. In retrospect, I wish I had challenged him more strongly about this, on moral grounds, because he was acting as if she had broken the deal that no one was allowed to change.

This couple's story is a good example of how an unnecessary divorce at one stage can turn into a necessary divorce later on. The wife was justified in leaving, in my view, because the marriage had become emotionally unbearable. I don't want to oversimplify this case because their problems reflected personal vulnerabilities on both their parts as well as a traditional male attitude toward a wife who pursues her personal goals. But the marriage became unbearable partly because the husband became a dissatisfied marital customer and chronic complainer.

When I contend that most divorces are unnecessary, what I mean is that one or both spouses could have turned it around by a change in attitude or behavior. Divorce is a last-ditch solution to marital problems that often could have been solved in less drastic ways, or at least adjusted to without injury to either party. But sometimes a spouse who does not want a divorce is forced into pulling the plug on the marriage because the other partner has reneged on his or her marital commitment through infidelity, chronic irresponsibility, or physical abuse. Other times the overt problems are not this serious, but the other spouse, sometimes coming from a sense of consumer entitlement, wages a steady emotional war until what had been an unnecessary and preventable divorce now becomes necessary and unavoidable. I remember a couple where the husband decided that his wife was holding back his growth and trying to control him. He began acting like an adolescent again. Over a period of two years, he engaged an escalating pattern of rages and long withdrawals during which he would not speak to his wife, punctuated by ever briefer periods when he was civil and supportive. He refused all offers to do marital therapy or to get personal help. Finally, his wife could not take it any longer and gave him an ultimatum to work on making their marriage better or leave. He left. Was she justified in ending the marriage? Yes. But it was like a proper decision to end life support for a patient that should never have been allowed to get this sick in the first place. The husband's consumer mind-set, probably combined with his personal crisis of middle age, turned an unnecessary divorce into a necessary one.

On a personal level, as my own marriage has endured for more than forty years now, I have come to value this kind of permanent bond more than when I was younger, even if it does not meet all of my needs or my wife's needs. A shared long life, starting out young and then growing old together, having birthed and nurtured children into adulthood, and the start of their own families makes the rewards of a long-term committed marriage surpass those of any other kind of relationship. The paradox here is that you get these rewards only when you don't keep focusing on the rewards. Remember Bea Arthur's line, "Don't look for happiness . . . it will only make you miserable."

Starting in the 1990s, in my writings for other therapists, I began to point out the therapeutic bias toward individual satisfaction as against family responsibilities and obligations. Gradually I began to listen differently to people's justifications for ending their marriages. I came to hear them like customer complaints, like someone explaining why they want to trade in a car for a new model, sell a house, or get rid of an old coat. Again, I recognize that people can become genuinely distressed about personal dissatisfactions in their marriage. But these new reasons often come down to saying that my psychological needs are not getting met in my marital lifestyle or that my mate is not doing an adequate job of meeting my needs.

There is another paradox here, because I also believe in advocating for oneself in marriage. Each spouse has genuine human needs to be treated with love, fairness, and respect. Being a patsy for a spouse's manipulation is not good for the marriage or oneself. When your spouse tries to control what you think or feel, you have to assert your boundaries. When your spouse treats you unfairly, you have to speak up. When your spouse fails to follow through on agreed-upon responsibilities, you have to confront him or her. These are all things I believe as a marital therapist, and they are not examples of consumer marriage.

Consumer marriage enters the picture when I focus mainly on what I am not getting in the marriage and on how my mate is not meeting my needs. I am in consumer mode when I fail to look at my own limitations, when I continually compare my spouse or marriage to my fantasies of other relationships, when I confuse my desires with my needs, when I lose the distinction between behavior that is completely unacceptable (such as physical abuse, infidelity, alcoholism, emotional cruelty, and chronic lying) and behavior that bothers me or saddens me (such as a spouse not giving me enough affection or emotional support, working excessive hours, showing lack of sexual interest, or having certain unlikable personality characteristics). The consumer attitude turns marital disappointments into marital tragedies and constructive efforts for improvement into entitled demands for change.

Here is a consumer marriage that ended in an unnecessary divorce: Sidney, recently retired and in a new second marriage to a woman in the prime of her career, dwelt continually on her work commitments and lack of availability to him. Like all couples, they had personal and relational difficulties that complicated their marriage, but what killed their relationship was the fact that Sidney became an increasingly disgruntled and resentful customer for his wife Mary's time and services. Although Mary did not start out speaking in consumer terms, she eventually did so by announcing that it was not in her best interests to jeopardize her career goals for a shaky marriage. This was a particularly sad ending to marital therapy, because neither really wanted to end the marriage, but the forces of individual self-interest finally overwhelmed their commitment.

Again, I want to stress that most people who are considering ending their marriages for what I term soft reasons are genuinely distressed and in pain. When we expect our needs to be met by others, we can be mightily frustrated when they don't come through.

The bar of our frustration tolerance gets lower and lower, and as good consumers, we look outside of ourselves for where the change should come from—namely, from our spouse. (I recall the words of one of my early supervisors, Charlie Seashore, who said that many marriages reach the point where one or both spouses say, "Someone around here has got to grow, and I'll be damned if it will be me.") When this attitude is combined with the inevitable personal vulnerabilities and baggage we bring into marriage, the glue does not hold.

Early in my career, all I needed to support a decision to end a nonabusive marriage was the statement that the marriage was now a source of pain and disappointment and that the love was gone. What I now see more clearly is that this pain and distress often come after years of dwelling on what one is not getting from the marriage, of complaining about the spouse's failings, of listening to the spouse defend and criticize back, of comparing one's marriage to other imagined relationships, and of gradually becoming more distant and resentful. In other words, after years living in a consumer marriage. A sense of personal entitlement to a high-quality marriage leads us to a focus on what is wrong with the other person, which leads to more things going wrong, and eventually to misery, which justifies leaving.

The Consumer Marriage at Home

Now we get to the most personal part: how the consumer culture affects our own marriages. It is impossible to live in American society without absorbing a good dose of the consumer culture of marriage. The problem with courtship is that it appears to fulfill the promise of consumer marriage. So when we start to realize, "Hey, this is getting to be a lot of work!" many of us find our minds invaded by consumer thoughts and confusions. A TV commercial showed a couple running a restaurant and the wife saying, in a soft, almost romantic tone of voice, that running a family business "is a lot like marriage—a little work and a lot of love." Wrong about business and wrong about marriage, both of which take a lot of work.

In long-term marriages, consumer thinking insinuates itself in a number of different ways. First is when we realize that the deficiencies in our mate or our marriage are not likely to go away. A couch-potato husband realizes that his wife is not going to become less busy after the children leave home; she just transfers her attention to community projects. A wife realizes that getting older is not softening some of her husband's opinionated hard edges or reducing the frequency of his bouts of depression. Her moodiness does not get better after menopause. His obsessive worrying does not diminish after he retires; he just transfers it from his job to their money situation. She loosens up a bit over the years in their sexual relationship, but their love life is never going to be the "hang from the chandeliers" kind that he once dreamed of. He requires a reminder each year about her birthday, despite past tears and apologies when he would forget.

The second main time that consumerism manifests itself is after the couple has tried hard to make changes, say, in a marriage education experience or in therapy. Surely, we hope, a good course of personal or marital therapy will shape up my mate. Although often there is positive change from these experiences, the leopards we marry don't often change their spots—or they change the wrong spots. Even if I see that I too contribute to the problems or limitations of my marriage, at some point in midlife I will probably face the reality that this relationship, the one we created together, has some built-in negative patterns that are here to stay. It's kind of like living with your own body for many decades; you know which parts are going to continue to creak and let you down.

Therapy and marriage education can help us change what we can change in ourselves and our relationships, but they can be dangerous if they set up the expectation that we should be rid of the flaws and painful parts of our marriage. (I am saying here in secular terms what the great religions of the world teach about human life.) At the end of therapy I often tell couples that their core strengths and core weaknesses will always be with them. The trick is to build on the strengths and contain and soften the impact of the weaknesses when they show themselves, especially in times of stress.

The third way that consumer thinking shows up in long-term marriages is when there is a change in how one of the spouses functions. I think of a couple, married thirty years, in which the husband had always wanted his wife to be involved in physical activities with him—biking, kayaking, and hiking. She complied with his wishes as a good sport, and for the good of the marriage, until she developed back problems that gave her an unarguable excuse to stop doing things she had not enjoyed. He couldn't quite blame her for saying "no," but he suspected (rightly) that she was not motivated to get her back into the kind of shape that would allow her to join him again in these activities. He was now a solo exerciser for the first time. This is a critical time for their relationship because the husband runs the risk of feeling sorry for himself and seeing his wife as a lesser provider of marital services. These feelings can set him up for temptation. More serious problems can occur when one of the spouses comes down with a chronic illness that seriously affects his or her ability to give to the other spouse. A marriage based mainly on consumer expectations will not survive.

The fourth consumer path is the way of comparisons. In the consumer model, we are always looking for newer and better models, even if we are basically satisfied with the one we have. The economy is based on comparisons between the good and the better. The latest computer chip will give me double the computer power of the last one. Who cares that what I have now is adequate? The most vibrant parts of the economy are based on quick obsolescence. In marriage, the temptation is always present to compare your current spouse with a prospective one, especially when you are upset with your spouse. Even if you have no intention of pursuing another relationship, the consumer virus of "comparisonitis" is an insidious one. A coworker, the spouse of a friend, a neighbor—anyone you get to know who has qualities that appear more attractive than your mate's—is a candidate for obsessing about how unfortunate you are for being married to the inadequate one you chose.

The danger here is not just that we compare and fantasize—that is normal, human, and probably unavoidable. I remember a young family medicine intern who told a support group, with some embarrassment, that when she examined a very fit young man, she found herself attracted to him and wishing that her husband took care of himself the way this man did. The problem is not these passing thoughts, feelings, and fantasies. The danger is when we allow ourselves to dwell on these comparisons and tell ourselves how sad it is that we are living with someone who offers us less than we deserve. Of course, we generally have little clue about what this person would actually be like as a spouse, and whether any supposed advantages over our current mate in some areas would be dramatically offset by disadvantages in other areas. The extremely fit guy might also be extremely narcissistic and also expect you to have the same body beautiful that he does.

Cheryl, the woman having the affair, fell into three of these patterns of consumer thinking. She focused on her husband's limitations as an unexciting partner and on the blandness of her long marriage, and she did not look at her own contribution. She convinced her husband to do therapy with her several times over the years, but little changed in the area of her core concerns. This convinced her that the marriage could not be improved, leaving her a disgruntled consumer. When she allowed herself to be kissed by a new man, she went into a frenzy of comparisons, fueled in large part by her prior preoccupation with what she was missing in her marriage. She was like someone on a desert island where a bottle of ice-cold Coke suddenly drops from the sky. (Maybe intoxicating beer would be more appropriate.) She was unable to evaluate the new relationship realistically because she felt so thirsty for something new. And with both her husband and her lover, she was taking the consumer attitude of concentrating on what the other person was providing her or not providing her. One made her feel safe but passionless by tucking her into bed at night, and the other lit her fire.

CONSUMER MARRIAGE QUIZ: IS YOUR MARRIAGE BECOMING A CONSUMER MARRIAGE?

How much consumer thinking has slipped into your marriage? Answer the questions below.

1. I (often, sometimes, rarely) compare my spouse unfavorably to others.
2. In relation to our problems, I (often, sometimes, rarely) dwell on my spouse's deficiencies; not my own.

3. I (often, sometimes, rarely) concentrate on how my spouse is not meeting my needs rather than how I am not meeting my spouse's needs.

4. I (often, sometimes, rarely) keep score: I add up when I do good things or when I think my spouse does something bad.

5. I (often, sometimes, rarely) think that my spouse is getting a better deal in this marriage than I am.

6. I (often, sometimes, rarely) focus on my spouse's defects rather than on his or her strengths.

7. I (often, sometimes, rarely) wonder whether I should have held out for someone better when I chose a mate.

8. When we have hard times, I (often, sometimes, rarely) ask myself whether the effort I am putting into this marriage is worth it.

If most of your answers are "rarely," congratulations. You do not treat marriage like a car that you can trade in when it ages and develops a touch of rust. If most of your answers are "sometimes," ask yourself whether things that you want are disguising themselves as things that you absolutely need. Try discussing your spouse's needs and wants. If three or more of your answers are "often," consumerism has severely infected your view of marriage. Do you want to be a "citizen" of your marriage, or take a "tourist visa" to travel the way of fantasy?

From *Take Back Your Marriage* (2nd ed.). Copyright 2013 by William J. Doherty.

Beyond these four general patterns of consumer thinking and attitudes in marriage, here is a list of specific thoughts and confusions that carry the musical themes of consumer marriage. I invite you to consider whether some of these tunes enter your mind at times.

• *"I am not getting my needs met!"* Turning wants into needs is what drives a market-based economy. Color TV was once a want and is now a need. Same with smartphones. In the early years of my marriage, I confused a need for my wife to be supportive of my academic work interests with a want or desire for her to be personally interested in what I was interested in. When I confused my legitimate need for someone to listen and even cheer me on at times with a more narcissistic desire to have a mate who was my clone, I put unfair pressure on Leah. I eventually got over this by reminding myself that my wife did not have to meet all my wants, and could not in any event. Discerning core needs from optional wants is a central task of resisting consumer marriage.

• *"I deserve better!"* Turning wants into needs leads to preoccupation with the sense of entitlement to something that we are not getting in our marriage. Of course, we are entitled to certain things from our mate, such as commitment, sexual fidelity, freedom from abuse, love, good will, and basic fairness. But once the list of entitlements gets too long or detailed, we begin to feel like an entitled victim of our marriage. If I had dwelled on being entitled to a spouse who was enthusiastic about my intellectual passion of the moment (these interests actually change so often that I don't know how that would be possible), then I would have hurt my marriage by feeling sorry for myself and resenting my wife. I have seen many spouses—wives, in particular—who work themselves out of their marriage by focusing on feeling that they're entitled to a mate who is warm, fuzzy, and able to share feelings on demand. Similarly, I have known many spouses—husbands, in particular—who justify their affairs on the basis that their mate is not sexually responsive enough. It's a slippery slope.

• *"If only I were married to that one!"* As discussed earlier, we never know what it's like to be married to someone other than the person we are with. If you find yourself dwelling on thoughts that someone else you meet or know has better marriage qualities than your current spouse, you are thinking like a misguided consumer. It may be that this person has certain traits in more abundance than your mate—smarter or more self-aware or better looking. But what you can't know is the downside that is revealed only in the furnace of married life—when smarter becomes patronizing or self-aware becomes self-obsessed or better looking becomes morbid fear of wrinkles. How do you resist comparing spouses? What most people do is to think positive thoughts about their partner and remind yourself that this is the one they are committed to and that they really know little about the other's mate potential.

- *"My marriage is not as good as your marriage."* This is a variation on comparing spouses. When you see other couples who look happy and in love, do you ever feel envious of their marriage? If you dwell on this thought, you are likely to unnecessarily devalue your own marriage. I have worked with many couples who looked wonderful on the outside and were miserable on the inside. I remember a couple confessing their embarrassment at the effusive praise for their marriage at their twenty-fifth wedding anniversary celebration. Guests said they envied this marriage. No one there knew that they had not made love for two years and were constantly bickering when alone. In fact, no one knows, except the couple and maybe their marital therapist, what goes on in the heart of another marriage.

- *"My spouse is a flawed person."* As I said before, dwelling on this thought is a common consumer thought pattern, fed by entitlement, confusion of wants and needs, and unnecessary comparisons. Remember, as a good consumer, that if you trade this mate in for a new model, you get a different set of flaws. And ask yourself whether the flaws you perceive are fatal or just bothersome. One client's spouse did have the fatal flaw of being a pedophile who would not seek help. Out he went. Another's spouse was physically violent, would not seek help, and blamed everyone else for his anger. Out he went, too. But most spouse flaws are not this grave, and we can come to accept them and refocus our thinking and energy on the other person's positives. Andrew Christensen and Neil Jacobson built an important model of marital therapy around the theme of acceptance (see their book *Reconcilable Differences*). I know a woman who says she saved her marriage when she accepted the fact that her husband, although he loved her deeply, did not know how to comfort her when she was emotionally distressed. She decided she could use her friends for that, and when she stopped expecting him to be perfectly empathetic, he was easier to be around when she was upset because he was less frightened of doing the wrong thing. Acceptance has a way of bringing out the best in all of us.

- *"I'm the good guy here."* We all have a great capacity for self-justification. In a poll, approximately seventy-five percent of divorced people thought they had worked hard to save the marriage, and only twenty-five percent thought that their ex-spouse had worked hard.

Something does not add up here, since the ex-spouses were also part of the seventy-five percent group! The easiest way to play the game of consumer marriage is to focus on our own righteousness while downplaying our contributions to marital problems. Cheryl, the woman having the affair, did this. Because she was able to be passionate with her lover, the problem in her marriage could not have stemmed from her own failings; the fault must have been her husband's. This is like saying that because I am happy on vacation, my unhappiness at home must be your fault. Self-justifying thoughts prepare you for pulling back or exiting, but you will take your tendency to self-justify into your next relationship.

What can we do instead of being an entitled customer in our marriages? In Cheryl's case, she could have seen the exciting kiss as a wake-up call to look inward at her own contributions to her life dissatisfactions and to her empty marriage. When she decided to follow the call of a new romance, she focused instead on the thrill of the affair and the impossibility of her husband changing. The more difficult but responsible approach would be to risk telling her husband bluntly about her frustrations and then either working hard for change or learning to live with these limitations without feeling victimized.

Cheryl ultimately took back her marriage. She ended the affair and started working on her relationship with her husband. Not without sadness, though, about letting go of the dream of consumer paradise in a permanent love affair. An emotional crisis with one of her children also helped to rivet her attention back on her family. She regained her marital commitment when she saw what was at stake—a long-term marriage, a husband who loved her, children who depended on that marriage, and a community of people affected by the marriage. She had been focusing on what she was not getting from her marriage, what she was entitled to get, what flaws in her husband had created the gap, and how she would be happier with a new model of husband. In the end, she came to see that she held citizenship papers in her marriage and just a tourist visa in her affair.

The best way to keep the consumer culture from dominating your marriage is to see yourself as a citizen of your marriage, which is another way to say to be intentional, committed, and part of a community. Being a citizen of a marriage means taking responsibility to make things better and not just be passive, to value the marriage itself and not just your own interest in it, to struggle to make it better by naming problems and changing yourself first, to take the long view that values your history together as a couple over short-term pain and struggle, to accept the inevitable limitations and problems, to see how your marriage affects many other people in your world, and to hold on to the dream, never completely fulfilled, of a more perfect union.

3 Don't Lose Your Marriage to Your Kids

So far we have talked about the dangers of the "me-first" approach to marriage. Now we take a sharp right turn by talking about how a more loving and self-sacrificing stance toward family life—the "children-first" approach—is also a danger to your marriage. This will take some explaining.

In some ways it is necessary to put our children first. They are the most vulnerable and needy people in our homes. When you want to make love with your mate and your wet, hungry baby wakes up and starts crying—well, you know what you do next. When your teenage daughter is beside herself after just being dumped by her boyfriend, you put your spouse's bad day on hold and attend to your daughter. Kids also enrich our personal and marital lives with their love, their joy, and their openness to what is new in the world. On the other hand, you and your spouse perhaps used to dine alone at 8:30 P.M. with a bottle of wine, but once you had kids you rightly established a family dinner ritual closer to 6:00 P.M., and you probably now drink milk along with the kids.

Adjustments like this are natural and inevitable. But there is a difference between adjusting your marriage to meet your children's needs and losing your marriage to parenthood. I think of Dave and Deirdre, loving parents and empty spouses. Somewhere between their son's birth and age six, their kids became their whole world. It began with never getting a sitter for their baby. Their excuse was that they were living away from extended family and did not trust the local kids. This may make sense for newborn babies who need special care, but even then Dave and Deirdre could have looked for other responsible new parents to exchange sitting with on a weekend night. So they stopped going out on dates together.

When their child was old enough to stay awake into the evening hours and resist going to bed, the couple never set a bedtime for him. He stayed in their midst, absorbing their attention, until he fell asleep on his own and was carted off to bed. Soon afterward, the couple went to bed themselves, drained from the day's work of earning a living and caring for a child. Then their daughter was born, and the pace of parenting quickened, absorbing even the small snippets of couple conversation they had stolen when they had just one child. Dave and Deirdre were not unhappy with their lives. They were devoted parents and cooperative companions. They thought that's what marriage was about once you became a parent. Actually, Deirdre complained sometimes to her friends that Dave did not pay enough attention to her, but her friends assured her that he was just a typical husband and that no one has much of a marriage when the children are little.

Their family life became even more child centered when their son started playing soccer at age six. It turned out that he had talent, and his parents enjoyed watching him play. Before long, they enrolled him on a more competitive team, a traveling team that practiced three times a week (four times during school breaks), plus home or away games every weekend. Tournaments were extra. Dave and Deirdre liked interacting with the other parents. The frequent practices meant that now they did not have family dinners very often, and the weekend travel, combined with their day jobs, meant that most weekends were pretty frantic. When their daughter, Denise, reached soccer age, she too joined the frenetic family pace, and now Dave and Deirdre frequently found themselves on separate soccer fields watching different kids. Dinner was a sandwich eaten in the car. Denise was not interested in a traveling soccer team, but she did sign up for competitive dance, which, it turned out, was as time consuming as soccer.

Dave and Deirdre had a typical middle-class family in today's world, revolving around the parents' work schedules and the children's activity schedules. They reflect the phenomenon of "helicopter parents" who are preoccupied with their children's safety and success in a competitive world. I wrote about this in 1999 in my book *Take Back Your Kids,* and in recent years there has been a flurry of books and magazine articles on the problem. Child psychiatrist Alvin Rosenfeld coined the term "hyper-parenting" to call attention to the tendency of today's parents to overfunction as parents and raise children who underfunction in the tasks of childhood, such as forging their own peer relationships and discovering their own interests and goals. Not enough attention, however, has been paid to the effects of hyper-parenting on marriage.

Notice that for Dave and Deirdre there was no couple schedule. At home, nearly all of their conversations center on the children or household logistics. Dave and Deirdre love each other, and sometimes talk about worries or stresses from their work or about the failing health of his father and her mother. But these conversations, like all their couple interactions, get interrupted constantly by the children. The parents could not imagine asking their children to refrain from interrupting a couple conversation. Nor could they imagine requiring their children to get to bed at a certain hour so the parents could have some off-duty time to relax together. Although they do get babysitters now, their occasional evenings out are with friends or to see a movie—not to spend time in quiet, personal conversation where they might reconnect emotionally. And their sex life, as you might imagine, is pretty stale at this point. It takes more than being good parents to keep intimacy alive.

If you think Dave and Deirdre have a challenge, what about Marc and Liz, a remarried couple with her kids living with them and his visiting every other week? Like many remarried couples, Marc and Liz have great difficulty making their relationship a priority without alienating the children. During week one, Marc tries to get some time with Liz in the evening, but her children insist she help them with their homework after they return from soccer practice. She feels torn between her husband and her children and chooses to spend the time with her children because she believes they need her more. During week two, when Marc's kids are with them, he is a full-time parent to them, scheduling himself every evening for their events and being available to them every minute otherwise. When Liz complains that he is not a husband during these weeks, he responds that he only has his kids every other week. And all along, the children are developing a sense of entitlement to their parent's time and attention and would raise a great stink if the couple acted like they were married lovers. Marc and Liz's situation is more challenging to their marriage than Dave and Deirdre's because in remarriages a spouse's time spent separately with his or her children feels more distancing to the other spouse than in a first marriage where the children belong to both parents equally.

Why Do We Give Away Our Marriages to the Kids?

In a two-parent family, marriage is the foundation of the family, the base of the family pyramid. It's the core relationship that preceded the children and the parent–child relationship. We fall in love with each other before we fall in love with our kids. After they leave home, we will still have each other, or so we hope. Our children rely on the stability and security of our marriage for their own stability and security. We all know these things; I am not writing rocket science here. So why do so many of us, like Dave and Deirdre, resign from being spouses when we become parents?

Part of the reason is that many of us do not know how to build our marriages after the newlywed period. That's what we discussed earlier: we get in our canoe and let the river take us south. But there is more involved when we are raising children. Children are natural and eager consumers of whatever time, attention, and goods and services that parents will provide. It's the job of parents to discern how much is enough, how much is too much, and to enforce the difference. Most parents nowadays understand this when it comes to providing material goods to children. Spoiling kids with material things is a cultural no-no except for buying them electronics, which seems to have no limits these days. But setting limits on how much time and attention we give them, and how many opportunities and activities we provide, is not stressed in our culture. Children nowadays own their parents. In a swift turn of a generation or two, we went from the norm that children should be seen and not heard when adults are around, to the norm that it is only the children who should be seen and heard when adults are around.

Take the case of bedtime. Dave and Deirdre are typical parents of young children in this arena. Studies are showing what many of us have observed: that bedtimes are vanishing from the family scene once kids get old enough to voice a strong preference. Some working parents say that they want to spend as much evening time as possible with their children, so they let them stay up as late as they want, until they fall asleep on their own. (Of course, children are then tired in the morning for school, and the parents are also losing the potential of good bedtime rituals with their children.) But there are other reasons harder to own up to. How do you make your child do something that he or she does not want to do? Why deal with the fuss and hassle of enforcing a bedtime routine? Suppose they keep getting up anyway? No, it's easier to simply let them watch TV or play a video game.

When I first came across this scenario, I thought I had entered a different culture. When I was growing up, we had fixed bedtimes that grew later as we got older. I still remember when I was old enough to start watching the *Ed Sullivan Show,* which came on at 8:00 P.M. For a couple of years, I could only watch the first half-hour, and then, finally, the whole show! If I had had my way, of course, I would have chosen my own bedtime; I fussed sometimes, but I complied.

When Leah and I had our own children, born in 1973 and 1975, we never considered not having bedtimes for them. The earliest bedtime I remember, when they were very young, was 7:30 P.M., followed for many years by 8:00 P.M., and then increasing until junior high. When they became teenagers, they determined their own bedtimes, with consultation from us if they appeared to be getting tired. I was usually in charge of the bedtime ritual, which began with baths thirty minutes in advance of the appointed time, followed by bedtime talks or books and a good-night kiss. Once they reached school age, we did not require lights out; they could read or play quietly until they were sleepy. But they could not leave their rooms or make requests of us, unless there was something important. We were off duty as parents.

Looking back, I can see three important functions of the Doherty bedtime arrangement. It gave the children down time and enough sleep. It gave us a chance to have a one-to-one ritual with each child; bedtime talks are some of my fondest memories as a parent. And it gave me and Leah adult time. It's not that we generally spent all of that time interacting, but at least we had the house to ourselves as a couple.

I first discovered the collapse of family bedtime routines a few years ago when doing marital therapy. I was working with a couple who had very little spark between them beyond regular skirmishes over chores and childrearing. I asked them how much time they spent together as a couple. Practically none, they reported. They never went out alone together, although they did see their extended families quite often. I asked if they had any time together after the children's bedtime. They looked at me with disbelief. Bedtime? They didn't know children who had fixed bedtimes. I felt as if I was now doing cross-cultural counseling. This couple had never established bedtime routines with their children and could not imagine doing so now that the kids were ten and twelve. The nightly pattern was that the wife was the first one in the house to go to bed, followed by the ten-year-old, the twelve-year-old, and the father. I never established whether the kids tucked the mother in, but I know that the husband did not.

How does this common bedtime scenario fit the idea of consumer parenting? Parenting has become like operating a twenty-four-hour, seven-day-a-week store, with service on demand. Of course, parenting has always been a full-time job, but nowadays it's not just being on call for children's core needs, but being ready to respond instantly as if to a customer in your store. When children are little, they want constant face-to-face time with you as a parent, or at least they want you in the next room and available to meet their needs, wants, and whims (which, to young children, are indistinguishable). When they become mobile teenagers, they now want you to be on a twenty-four-hour cell-phone or instant-message leash in case they require information or permission for some activity. I hear parents complaining that their teenager scolds them when their cell phone is turned off. Who, you might ask, are the parents, and who are the children?

On the home scene, children of all ages now have a new universal human right to interrupt adult conversation at any time and for any reason. The adults must disengage from their conversation and turn immediately to the child. Many parents now define rudeness, not as a child interrupting willy-nilly for a minor reason that could wait, but as adults putting the child off while finishing their sentence! It would be rude to keep talking or to ask the child to say "Excuse me" and request permission to interrupt. Can you imagine telling your seven-year-old, who wants an answer now about tomorrow's swimming outing, to wait until you and your spouse finish talking about something? If you can, you are already resisting the pull of consumer parenting. If you can't imagine it but would like to, you are on your way.

WHO OWNS YOUR MARRIAGE—YOU OR YOUR KIDS?

It's easy to find reasons why your kids' needs are front and center, but if you neglect your spouse in the process of parenting, you won't be doing your kids any favors. If you read these statements and answer "yes" more than three times, you're giving away your married life to your kids and should work to set up boundaries to get back a life with your mate.

1. Five nights out of seven, your preadolescent kids go to bed whenever they want, and it's usually well after 9:00 P.M.

2. When you've finally found a moment with your spouse, even if it's in the car on the way to the soccer match, your kids invariably ask you to turn up the music, give them a juice box, or demand you hear about the latest video game, and you find it easier to listen than to ask them to wait until you're done talking with your spouse.

3. You haven't had a night out alone together in a month—and you can't even remember the last one before that.

4. The lock on the bedroom door is growing rusty with disuse.

5. Your down time as a couple is always family time, for example, spent watching a Disney video with the kids instead of listening to jazz on the deck while the kids watch the movie indoors.
6. When the choice at the moment is between talking to your spouse about his or her day, or playing ball with your kids, and you almost always choose the kids.
7. When you've finally finished driving the kids to violin lessons and swim practice and have completed that science project you just found out was due tomorrow and your spouse wants to sit down and relax with you, you just can't resist working on building Tanya's dollhouse "while we talk."

Your Children Will Have Mixed Feelings

I have to warn you that your children will not immediately like the change if you decide to take your marriage back from their consumer demands. Who can blame them? Who would not want a servant on continual call? And who would not resent it when the servant suddenly decides to have a life? I hope you understand that I am not talking about neglecting one's children—although they may think so at first—but about creating a balanced family life that allows for a marital relationship to prosper. Deciding to take your child out of traveling soccer because the toll is too great on your family and couple time will not win you a popularity contest with your child and may bring criticism from other parents. To support parents in making these decisions, I helped to start an initiative called "Putting Family First." (You can learn about it on the Web at *puttingfamilyfirst.org*.) Getting a handle on children's outside activities is essential for creating family balance, which in turn is essential for a marriage to flourish.

Starting bedtime routines for your disgruntled children will take perseverance. Telling your junior high schooler that you are available to help with homework only until 8:30 P.M., and that you are off duty afterward, will at first seem selfish to your child. Telling your daughter that you and her stepfather are going away for the weekend and that you will get someone to drive her to her soccer game may elicit protests from her (your new marriage is not high on her priority list) along with opposition from other soccer parents who will think you are neglecting your daughter by not appearing on the sidelines.

If your children have learned that their desire for attention always trumps your marriage, then you will have to be patient with their complaints as you make the shift. Tell them why you are asking them to take what feels like second place for periods of time. Tell them you need date nights because you like each other and need to spend time together. Don't apologize for creating more balance. Invite their support as citizens of the family, not just as unhappy customers of your services. Be firm about changes you make. Don't backtrack when they resist, but make reasonable compromises; for example, have a time for their bedroom door to be closed but not necessarily for lights to be out, let your child play on the nontravel soccer team, or promise your five-year-old that you will read a book to her every night before your couple time.

If you believe in these changes, and give your children clear reasons related to your couple time, they will eventually come to value the shift in the family environment. And if you start when your children are young, they will accept the need for family balance from the beginning. When our youngest was about four years old, Leah and I established a couple talk ritual after dinner. I will describe this more fully later when we discuss talk rituals, but for now the point is that we taught our children to leave us alone for fifteen minutes after dinner every night while we talked about our day and what was on our minds. We had to remind them occasionally to hold off on interrupting unless there was something urgent, but mostly they cooperated. Years later, I asked our grown daughter how she felt as a child when we sent her off to play while we had our coffee time. She said she remembered feeling "safe." She felt comforted that we took time together every night, more secure because we were being a couple. I recall the same feeling when my own parents had tea together in the kitchen at night, talking quietly. Something about my world felt safe.

Strategies for Not Losing Your Marriage to Your Parenting

I'd like to pull together my suggestions for the tricky task of being terrific parents in a terrific marriage. Making your marriage a priority does not mean neglecting your children. As in the rest of life, it's a matter of balance. But for most of us, the harder side of the seesaw to put weight on is our marriage. Kids are better at advocating for time and attention than we are as spouses.

- If you are married, remind yourself repeatedly that your marriage is the foundation of your family and the cornerstone of your children's security. It is primary, not secondary, for everybody's well-being. This is not to say that children cannot prosper in a single-parent family (many do), but that in a married, two-parent family the foundation is the marriage. When it goes sour, the family goes sour. A lot of research on two-parent families shows that good marriages lead to good parenting and that conflicted marriages lead to bad parenting.

- Remind yourself repeatedly that your children are apt to be better fighters for their needs—nature has programmed them to be good at getting our attention—than you and your mate are at fighting for the needs of your marriage. You've got to lean toward your marriage in order to have balance between your marriage and your children.

- Limit your family's outside activities so that you have two rare elements for today's families: time to hang out as a family and time to hang out as a couple.

- Have fixed bedtimes for your children, after which you are off duty and can be alone as a couple.

- Don't let your children interrupt every conversation you have. If you really want to finish something, or if one of you needs a supportive listener, feel free to politely ask your children to come back later after you have finished talking. And teach them to ask if they can interrupt.

- For some important couple conversations, tell your children that you are going to your bedroom to talk and that you would like them not to interrupt you unless something important happens, such as someone being hurt.

• Limit the amount of time you devote to your children's school homework every night. Teachers complain that some well-educated parents do not let their children learn on their own. Unless your child has special learning problems, do not routinely devote your whole evenings to being a tutor, in part because you will have no time for yourself and for your spouse.

• Carve out private time for yourselves as a couple. Even a fifteen-minute period is wonderful if you do it every day. This might be over coffee after dinner, as my wife and I have done, or after putting the children to bed. When your children are old enough, you can go for an after-dinner walk around the neighborhood.

• Carve out private space. Consider letting your children know that your bedroom is private when your door is closed and that they should knock. This sends the message that there are certain marital things that children do not share in without checking.

• Get sitters and go out on regular dates. This is not only good for your relationship, but it also sends your children the message that indeed you are a couple who do special things together: you dress up, look great, and go out for a good time together. Whatever their protests, even young children can handle a few hours of separation from their parents. Older children may be glad to be rid of you if they have good babysitters (our children used to suggest we go out so they could see their favorite babysitter), and they will feel more secure because they sense that you enjoy each other's company. Adolescents will be impressed that old-timers like you still date.

• Never complain about your spouse to the children. This tells your children that your primary relationship is with them, not with your spouse. Here I am referring to important complaints about your mate's personality or character, not the occasional frustrations, say, about being late or forgetting to turn the lights off.

• If you have a heated argument in earshot of the children (sometimes it's unavoidable), then let them see you be affectionate when you've made up. This helps children know that your relationship is strong enough to recover from anger and misunderstanding, and that you are taking care of your marriage. You can check out with your children if they feel upset about your arguing. During a bedtime talk, I once asked my daughter, when she was about seven, whether she felt upset when she heard her mother and me argue. I will never forget her reply: "No, it doesn't bother me, because I know you are not going to get a divort." (That was her word for "divorce.") I told her she was right about that.

• When your children are old enough, and if you can afford it, get away for an occasional weekend together without the children. This is a way to revive your marriage.

• Be open with your children about what you are doing for your marriage, and why you are doing it. You don't have to give lectures, but make sure your children know that you are setting limits on attention and availability for them because you love each other and want to make sure you stay close. Your explanations, of course, will be different for children at different levels of development, but all children past the toddler stage can understand that you like each other and like to be alone and do things together sometimes. With adolescents, there are moments when you can quietly share your philosophy of marriage. I did with my kids, and it's gratifying to see that they share these values in their own marriages.

The Marriage-Centered Family

I have known only a handful of people over the years who made their marriage such a singular priority that they neglected their children. These were fairly self-centered couples who should probably not have had children. So I am not especially worried about married people taking my message wrong when I talk about a "marriage-centered family." The greater danger for most of us is to lose our marriage to the demands of parenthood rather than losing our kids to the demands of our marriage (although this happens sometimes in stepfamilies). In a two-parent family, we either fight to create and keep a marriage-centered family, in which the couple relationship is the stable fulcrum of the family and the couple together care for their children, or we become a child-centered family in which the marriage goes on the shelf. Marriages can safely go on the shelf for spurts of time without damage, such as when a child is sick or an elderly parent needs respite from the demands of caregiving. But when marriages stay on the shelf for extended periods, they wither and dry, becoming unrecognizable when we eventually retrieve them.

A friend of mine whose daughter just went off to college told me that several of her daughter's new college friends had just heard shocking going-away news from their parents: that the parents' marriages were over now that the last child was launched. Don't think this is not a big crisis for an eighteen-year-old. The greatest danger of having a child-centered family is that, when the children leave home, so does your marriage. It's like not using one of your arms for twenty or more years. You lose it. No one wants this when they get married, but the currents are swift after children come into our lives. It's not that children inevitably divide us; in fact, children can provide additional glue for marital commitment. It's that caring for them in today's world, if we are not intentional about our relationships, tends to decrease our attention to nurturing our marriages. Hyper-parenting comes at a price.

The second danger is that, even if we stay together after the children leave home, we are permanently diminished as couples. We choose vital parenthood but devitalized marriage. Not as a conscious choice, but because we focused our energy, attention, and creativity only on our children's needs to the neglect of the needs of our marriage. Our marital light never recovered its brightness. Many people say they are fine with this, but I can't believe that this was their first choice when starting out their lives together.

The third danger is the most benign, but is still regrettable. We re-find our marriage after the children leave. The light shines bright again. This outcome is positive, but it's also sad for two reasons: the many years of unmet marital potential and the lack of good marital role models for our children. I also worry about these couples' staying power when their health declines, because they do not have a track record of being able to focus on their relationship when there is another big demand on their energy and attention.

I don't hold out my own marriage as a model for all couples. And I don't mean to imply that we had no struggles with our children, or made no mistakes. We had our share of both. But I know we did one thing well: we taught our children that we valued our marriage without devaluing them, that more for us meant more for them, that we were mates before we were parents, and that in the solar system of our family, our marriage was the sun and the children the planets, rather than the other way around.

4 Take Back Time for Your Marriage

Here's one of the chief ironies about marriage today: If you still care deeply for each other, you probably feel starved for time together. The couples who don't wish for more time together are generally the ones who don't like each other much anymore. They are relieved to be apart. But many of us, especially when we are raising children and have busy jobs, live our marriages with a chronic sense of deficit about the time we spend together as a couple. Ironically, even when people are frustrated with their relationship, they often still want to spend more time together to see whether that will help them like their spouse more.

Why? Because the competitors for our daily time are far more assertive than we are about our marriages. We talked earlier about children, who at least are highly deserving competitors! Here we will be talking about four others: jobs, adult schedules, individual hobbies and recreational pursuits, and TV, personal electronic devices, and the Internet. Most of us surrender our marriage to a combination of these hungry, assertive life partners.

I mentioned feeling starved for marriage time. Generally one of the partners is feeling it more than the other, which leads to what my graduate school mentor Robert Ryder used to call "the common cold of marriage"—the pursuer–distancer cycle. Also termed the "demand–withdraw" pattern, it occurs when one spouse feels chronically more dissatisfied with the couple's level of connection and tries to get the other person to pay more attention and spend more time together. (It may be about other things than time—conversation and sex are common examples—but time is central to most of these patterns.) When the pursuer demands more time, the distancer feels threatened at the loss of independence and digs in his or her heels. The distancer not only does not give more time, but withdraws more emotionally. This scares the pursuer, who more forcefully demands increased time and connection. This in turn scares the distancer, who fears that compromise will result in giving in to unreasonable demands; so the distancer pulls further away.

Some version of this struggle over time is nearly universal in marriage. In heterosexual couples, the most common one is that the woman is the pursuer for more time together and the man the distancer. Most couples manage to contain this pattern before it becomes too destructive, but most never fully resolve it. Sadly, the distancer often would genuinely like more good time together, but in the struggle never gets to express that desire. Sadder still, many couples never look broadly at their lives to assess the competition for the marriage. They focus on one competitor, such as one spouse's job or the other's hobby, and never get the overall picture of what they are up against. Thus their strategies for change are simplistic and one sided: "If you would work less . . . play less . . . quit your committees . . . watch less TV, get off your iPhone, then we would have plenty of time for each other." The other responds, "If you would get off my back, we would get along quite well." The subtext is "You're the problem here, so it's up to you to change." Let's look together at the common competitors for marital time, and what we can do about them. Some of what follows may fit your experience, and some will not.

Love's Labor's Lost: The Demands of Work

Let's get to the extreme case first: some work schedules are incompatible with the kind of companionship and intimacy in marriage that most of us want. I remember realizing this for the first time when I was working with a married couple in their forties, who worked different shifts—she days and he nights. They barely overlapped thirty minutes a day. An occasional weekend day together they spent arguing and running errands. The only real conversation they had each week was when they saw me for therapy! I doubted that they could rebuild their shaky marriage with their current work schedules, and I told them so. They saw the problem, but their commitment at this point, in a rocky second marriage of two years' duration, was so low that neither wanted to jeopardize their job status by making a shift. They ultimately decided to divorce. You can't bind what don't cling. Some work schedules are incompatible with marriage, especially ones that need repair.

In less extreme cases, one spouse has a job with excessive hours and the other does not. When the first spouse comes home late, at least the other is there, available for connection. I think of a young mortgage broker who, during boom years for real estate, worked a hundred hours per week. Make hay while the sun shines, was his motto. He saw himself as doing this for his homemaker wife and their three-year-old daughter. Ideally, he would have preferred a fifty-hour-a-week job, but this was the career he had chosen. He reminded his wife of what his career brought them in terms of housing and lifestyle. She was lonely and starved for time with him. When she complained, he told her that he could not control the real estate cycle, and that when the work was there, he had to do it. He never told her that he missed her or wished their situation were different. When, in therapy, he did say these things—and I believe he meant it—she softened her demands because she felt more connected with him. He began to make more effort to call her during the day and to not work Sundays. Because this couple only stayed in therapy for a few sessions, I do not know what became of them. But I worry that they needed more serious change than they had achieved. Their marriage was held hostage to the husband's loyalty to the real estate cycle.

When we move from extreme workloads into the realm of everyday work demands, the challenge gets to be how the couple manage the almost inevitable competition between work and marriage. I see four common problems for couples when at least one has a demanding, but not impossible job.

- When work interferes with important family activities, such as dinner and bedtime rituals, and one spouse has to carry the load of evening responsibilities, it often creates distance in the marriage. In many cases, it would be better for your marriage to come home early for dinner and work at home after dinner, or substitute family breakfast for family dinner.

- When you can't count on being home at predictable times. Most spouses do not cope well with unpredictability. My advice is to use the telephone to be as predictable as possible. Let your mate know the minute something has changed your plans for being home. And express your regret. The biggest problem is feeling second fiddle to a spouse's work schedule. It can help a lot if the spouse with the greater work demands expresses regret and frustration about those demands, rather than treats them as natural and inevitable. Do you see the difference between just the facts—"I have to work later than I had expected because my replacement just called in sick; I'll get home when I can"—and "I'm really sorry that I won't be home for dinner; I'm frustrated that my replacement just called in sick; I'd rather be on my way home." Remember: for the most part, it's the feelings and not the time.

- When your work interferes with a big marital event, such as an anniversary or a birthday. I've worked with physicians who had to respond to an emergency on the night of their anniversary dinner. Again, the problem is more how you handle it than the interference itself. When you respond matter of factly or defensively ("Sorry, I gotta go to the hospital for an emergency; what can I do?"), your spouse's disappointment is compounded by the sense that it is no big deal to you because your work comes first. Instead, I advise pouring it on with your disappointment and apologizing profusely. (Men in particular have trouble doing this, if logically they know that it is not their fault.) And then make up for it in a big way. Reschedule the dinner yourself at a much fancier place, or upgrade your anniversary celebration to a weekend away. And get backup at work next time!

- When you are physically at home and psychologically at work. This was my biggest challenge for many years in my marriage. Being in academia, I could control my schedule. Being home for dinner was not a problem, nor was having to work according to a supervisor's schedule. My challenge was that I was often thinking about a work project or problem while I was in conversation with my wife or kids. This can be maddening for a spouse, harder even than having the other spouse gone at work. I eventually learned that brooding about work was not productive for work or family life. If I am preoccupied with a work problem, I am now more likely to verbalize that fact, rather than trying to pay attention to Leah and secretly thinking about work. Instead of trying to cut off the work-related thoughts, I started to notice when they were invading my home conversations, and tried to do something about it, such as saying, "I'm having trouble focusing tonight because I am worried about. . . ." A few minutes (just a few!) of direct conversation about what is stressing me often helps me be able to listen better to Leah. Strange to say for a practicing therapist, I had to learn that expressing what I am stressed about helps it go away, as long as I decide in advance to keep this sharing brief so that it does not dominate the evening.

For most married couples, the work of one or both partners is a major rival to the marriage because of the time it takes from the marriage. But couples throughout the ages have worked hard in life. The main problem is generally not the sheer number of hours worked but the feeling that the other's work is more important, emotionally and psychologically, than oneself. With this in mind, many of the adjustments do not require a drastic change in career, although in extreme cases that might be necessary for the sake of the marriage. Mostly they require thoughtfulness about preserving time for the marriage in the face of work demands. For example, one wife who generally worked some hours between dinner and bedtime (he preferred that she watch TV with him) decided to get up earlier in the morning to have a quiet breakfast with her husband. A business executive, upon realizing that his wife wanted a sense of being a priority on his schedule, picked up his cell phone during a marital therapy session, called his secretary, and booked his wife for a Thursday lunch (her best day) every week indefinitely. That wasn't the end of the adjustments they had to make, but it was an important beginning.

Overscheduling the Time of Our Lives

I remember Ann as committed to church activities as anyone in the parish. If there was a need, Ann would fill it. Most of these activities, of course, were on weekday evenings, which meant she was gone from home most evenings. Her husband was a busy professional person, but was home evenings with the children when she was gone. He worked late into the night after she got home. He was not a member of the church, or a believer. Can you see where this marital boat is heading? Affairs—hers with the church and his later with a colleague—ended the marriage.

We talked before about the overscheduling of children and youth. Here I address the same problem with adults. Not work scheduling, but scheduling ourselves into good activities in our communities, such as committees, volunteering, club memberships, and religious activities. All good, all involved in serving others. The problem is that when we have no counterbalancing schedule with our spouse, our individual schedules swallow the time for our marriages.

If most parents were not already overbooked with children's activities, perhaps the adult activities would not be such a concern. But in truth, between chauffeuring kids and being personally involved in two or three adult activities, you know what will come last in your life—your marriage. It's a function of what is scheduled and to whom we feel accountable for our time. We feel accountable to our children and the commitments we have made to and for them. We feel accountable to the book club we promised to attend monthly, to the religious education committee we joined, and to the fundraising committee of the PTA. But most of us do not feel accountable to have face-to-face time alone with our mate, because we never schedule it.

Our marriage gets what is left over on our schedules. Don't forget the pursuer–distancer pattern, which rears its head here. Your spouse may accept your work hours and your childrearing hours, but become resentful at your optional schedule of community activities. Dash home from work, grab sandwiches while transporting the kids to practice, rush home, change clothes, and then head to your committee meeting at your church or synagogue. Return home exhausted at ten o'clock to a spouse who is frustrated at you. Sounds like a life to me!

If your spouse joins you by overscheduling him- or herself too, you might feel relieved. Both of you collapse in front of the television at ten o'clock. But we know from research on marriage that when the pursuer stops trying to get more connection, the marriage is in serious trouble. When both parties have surrendered their active citizenship in the marriage, it may be over soon. Or it may go on automatic pilot for years, destination uncertain, but the Gulf of Mexico is a serious possibility.

I do not want to disparage community involvement. In some ways, we need more of it, not less. The issue is one of balanced priorities, and the need to schedule time for one's marriage. We also should develop ways for couples to be involved together in community and religious activities, so that giving to the community can also strengthen the marriage. Many years at our church my wife and I worked together to lead the fund-raising auction, something that helps our community and our marriage. One side benefit I have noticed is that people see us being a couple in public and relate to us that way in the future. The church becomes an asset to our marriage, and our marriage becomes an asset to the church. The other way in which community involvement can strengthen marriage is when each spouse openly supports and encourages the other's individual contributions. Building a good marriage does not mean owning one's mate, but rather creating a balance between internal nurturing and external nurturing of a community. I don't have any rules or prescriptions for finding this balance, but I can say that it requires continual monitoring and adjustments. One pattern Leah and I have found helpful is to think of seasons of greater involvement in community, followed by seasons of focusing more on home.

Individual Hobbies and Recreation

In the face of frantic family schedules, how do we add in individual hobbies and recreation without completely putting our marriages on hold? I have been struck over the years of working with couples by how readily husbands assume the right to their personal outside activities, while wives do not assert a similar right. Chuck's hunting weekends in the fall were not negotiable, the dates having been set by Chuck and his friends months in advance. Feeling burdened by being a single parent for four weekends during the busy fall, his wife, Sarah, assertively negotiated free afternoons the weekends in between Chuck's hunting weekends. She actually would have preferred that Chuck be home during fall weekends, and then she would not have felt she had to claim her own free time. But if he was going to be selfish, she thought, so would she.

Just as with work and community involvement, individual hobbies and recreation are usually not the problem in themselves. It's how they are decided on and how they are handled. Four weekends a year for a lifelong passion for hunting does not have to be troublesome for a marriage. But Chuck approached this as a personal entitlement, with the expectation that Sarah and the children would have to adjust. Sarah felt she had no choice but to yield, although with complaints and a negotiation of her own entitlement during the off weekends. Notice that these were individualistic plans. Neither Chuck nor Sarah advocated anything for the marriage to offset the individual activities.

How would a couple like this pull out of this pattern? Chuck would have to begin by not assuming next year that he will automatically schedule four weekends of hunting during the family's busy fall season. Hobbies and recreation have to be labeled as secondary to family and marriage priorities. Secondary does not mean off the schedule, but it means working around family and marriage priorities and being curtailed if necessary. Sarah would have to be honest about how she saw the hunting weekends fitting into family and marriage priorities. If four weekends seemed too much, she should say so directly. The keys to handling the emotional aspects of this conversation are to avoid assigning selfish motives to the other person and to avoid just caving in to the spouse's demands. With my help in therapy, Chuck and Sarah were able to have a low-key conversation on this perennial problem for the first time; no one was labeled selfish and no one resentfully went along. Later in this chapter, I describe ways you can help yourself and your mate manage these dilemmas.

If the joint decision is for a spouse to pursue the individual activity, then the next step should be for both partners to figure out how to offset the lost time. Chuck and Sarah both discussed how she can get some "off-duty" time during fall because of the overload when Chuck is gone. Since they both own the idea of Chuck pursuing his hunting hobby, they should both own Sarah getting some of her needs met. And then there are the marriage's needs and the children's needs. Chuck and Sarah brainstormed ways that they can make sure they connect as a couple during the fall, and also ways that the family can avoid feeling fragmented by tag-team parenting. For example, maybe the family can have a special meal on Sunday evenings when Chuck returns. Maybe the couple can have a special date night during the week before one of his trips. Maybe he cancels one weekend and the couple does a weekend trip.

The point is to avoid the consumer approach to individual hobbies and recreational interests. In consumer marriage, the spouses negotiate their individual preferences instead of collaboratively trying to see that they retain balance in their common life. In our culture, the consumer approach most often will mean that husbands get their way, because they are more likely to unashamedly assert what they want to do for themselves, whereas wives are more likely to want to make sure that everyone else's needs are satisfied before they get their own met. This imbalance breeds resentment in wives and guilt in husbands for being accused of selfishness. One alternative is at least a balance of entitlements; for example, younger wives nowadays are more assertive than their elders about going out with their friends. A better alternative is to take a citizenship approach, in which each straightforwardly brings needs and desires to the table in the context of what is good for the marriage and for each partner.

Reclaiming Time from E-Connections

Probably no time in human history has had so many distractions from conversation and connection. Television is an almost old-fashioned, low-end distractor in a world where we carry computers in our pockets that connect us instantly to people and information. Writer Linda Stone has coined the term "continuous partial attention" to describe the state of affairs in which we monitor an incoming stream of information from multiple sources so as not to miss anything—all the while missing connection with the person who is actually with us. This is different from traditional multitasking where we are trying to accomplish more than one thing at a time; it's a nervous way of staying in partial touch with many people lest we feel completely out of touch. Now that more than a third of U.S. adults own a smartphone (and two-thirds of them keep it next to their bed), we are going to have to heed social psychologist Sherry Turkle's admonition that we'd better figure out how to live with them and keep our relationships sound.

You've seen it. A couple sits at a restaurant for a dinner out, and one pulls out a smartphone either to answer a call or to check text messages or e-mail. The other eats for a while, then pulls out a device to do the same. Now the first person has little incentive to return to the conversation. And on they go. Increasingly, I don't pick up signals of irritation from either party at the other's distraction; it's just the nature of relationships nowadays. Every two-way conversation can be interrupted by hundreds of other people, or by a desire to know the score in a ball game or to answer a call from someone you talked to just a few hours ago. In Sherry Turkle's terms, we are "alone together."

I recently succumbed to the iPad when my university offered me one for free. It's a portable temptation to read anything on demand, whether the latest ball game score or the political gossip. My wife and I tease that we never have to exchange more than one sentence of disagreement about something factual because we can look it up so easily on the iPad. Not to mention how easy it is to get lost in a solitary pursuit of that newspaper article I heard about from a friend. Our solution to keeping it in its place is to put the charming little thing away in a basket unless we actually need it.

When it comes to TV, we know that the average household in the United States now has three television sets and that at least one of these sets is on most of the time when family members are home. But little research has been done on the impact of TV on marriage. I will tell you what I see.

Couples tell me that when they finally get their kids to bed, or chores done, they tend to collapse in front of the television set. Often one of the spouses has been there first, is watching a show, and may not want to be interrupted. When the other spouse starts talking, the TV watcher doesn't look that person's way and responds shortly. "Is there a problem?" the other asks. "No, I'm just trying to watch this show. Wait for a commercial." At the first moment of the day when the couple are alone, they have to wait for a TV commercial.

When no one is specifically sitting down to watch TV, having it on in the background leads to misunderstandings when one spouse starts to attend to the television while the two are talking. You thought you had your mate's attention, and then when you look up, his or her eyes and ears are on the set and he or she hasn't heard what you said. This happens to all couples at times; it's the nature of the in-and-out attention we pay to TV more than any other medium.

When the couple goes to bed, chances are there is a TV in the bedroom. In my view, that is one of the worst mistakes a married couple can make, because this invites the greatest household absorber of time and attention directly into the intimate sanctum of a marriage. I realize that the decision is an innocent one and that some couples relax together watching the news or Jay Leno, but they can do that on the couch in the living room. The bedroom, in my view, should be media free and thus open to couple connection through words and touch.

Then there's the being on the computer and the Internet. At least when your partner is sitting at a computer, you know where he or she is focused, unlike with the TV and smartphone, where you could be sitting together and then realize the other person is not with you. The downside is that the Internet is a powerful absorber of individual time and attention. Starting in the mid-1990s, therapists began to see couples in which one spouse spends all his or her free time gaming or doing social media on the Internet. For some couples, time on the Internet has replaced work hours as a main source of conflict. For other couples, the temptation of Internet affairs has become a serious problem, especially now that it is so easy to relocate old flames. As with all technology, it's not usually the Internet use that's the problem. It's what it means to the spouses and what else they are not doing.

Taking Back Your Time

Here I would like to pull together my take-home messages about marriage and time. I begin with how to see the big picture of time in your marriage and then move into specific recommendations that have worked for me and couples I have known in my work and personal life.

- If you are concerned about your own time away from your marriage and family, keep a log of your hours for a while. I did this once by looking at my last year's schedule of evening and weekend talks, plus travel. I readily saw that I was spending too much time on these activities for the good of my marriage and personal well-being, particularly during certain periods of the year. Do this assessment yourself and then share your findings with your mate, with ideas about change if necessary. Do not keep a log of your mate's activities, or that will seem like supervising. If you can't change your schedule immediately (as is often the case because of commitments made), then plan ahead for when you can start making different decisions. Once I realized that I was doing too many evening and weekend activities, I did not cancel any that I had agreed to, but I began to say "no" to many new invitations. I told my wife about each one, and about why I was doing it, so that she would know I was working on making changes and so that she could encourage me. It's not always easy to cut back, but the main thing is for me to let my wife know I am concerned about the effect of my work schedule on our relationship.
- Plan marital time. When I was in graduate school and working and raising babies, my wife and I had terrible schedules. So we decided to have a long breakfast out together every Friday morning and then hang out for a while. That weekly time helped us "cling" until we could straighten out our schedules.
- When other demands eat into your marital time, remind yourself of what you are missing and tell your spouse how bad you feel about that. As I keep saying, it's often the failure to express regret, and sometimes to apologize, that most often makes the other person feel like second fiddle.

- Use the time you do have better. It's not like most of us are using the full potential of the limited time we have. Later I will discuss this extensively under the heading of "marital rituals." You can improve your marriage a lot with small changes in your time schedules.
- Pursuers, avoid nagging about spending more time together. Bring up your concerns periodically, at a calm moment, in terms of your hopes for your marriage, rather than bringing them up continually and by criticizing your spouse's priorities.
- Distancers, ask yourself what you hope for in your marriage and what it will take to fulfill those hopes. Think proactively rather than defensively about finding more time for your marriage. And think creatively about better using the time you already have.
- Continuous partial attenders, develop ground rules with your mate about when you will check your messages and when the smartphone is at rest. Let the other person know at the outset of a conversation if you will have to interrupt for a message, and then return to full focus afterward.
- If you are married to a continuous partial attender who seems married to a device, bring up the issue at another time when you are not frustrated. That helps keep the conversation from generating into an argument about the most recent call or text. Instead, say that you like having time to be together alone without distractions and would like to figure out a way for that to happen more regularly, perhaps starting with times when you are out having a meal or taking a walk.
- When working on your time together, don't make the main issue the external time drainer—work, leisure activities, TV, the computer, or the cell phone. Instead focus on how to be more intentional with these external forces so that you can benefit from them and keep your relationship a high priority. I knew a young couple who argued consistently about the husband's commitment to weekend football on TV. It was only when they stopped arguing about football and TV, and listened to each other's needs for two things they both wanted—connection with each other and leisure time for things they loved—that they were able to solve the "football" problem.

• Use your social time with friends as a way to build your bond instead of creating separate silos. Individual friends are important, but it's best to build in time for them that does not take away from the limited time you and your mate have together. I've been having lunch monthly with my friend Patrick for more than twenty years, and we mostly do it during the work week. When I go for Saturday walks with my friend Mac, we try to find a time when we would not otherwise be doing something with our wives. On the other hand, socializing together as a couple with friends can build your relationship as long as it is not a substitute for alone time.

If all of the above does not work, you may have a big structural problem with your time use. In other words, you might have a lifestyle that is inconsistent with the kind of marriage you and your spouse want. If that is your conclusion, then I encourage you to consider a shift in career, hobbies, or some other absorber of your time and energy. Remember your wedding vow about "forsaking all others"? That might mean forsaking what drains your time and your mind. It's not only a sexual affair that threatens marriage. It can be a time or attention affair as well.

5 Resist Family and Friends Who Would Undermine Your Marriage

Unless you are very unlucky or have a vengeful ex-spouse, there is probably nobody in your life who would deliberately set out to hurt your marriage. But unintentional sabotage is common and, in some ways, more dangerous. Earlier we talked about how the "I deserve the best" consumer culture sends messages that can erode our commitments to marriage. Here we discuss how particular people in our lives can undermine our commitments because they are also influenced by the same forces. I am not encouraging paranoia about people being out to get you. Research studies over the past fifteen years have shown how family and friends can contribute to the quality of a marriage by supporting the relationship and being a marriage-friendly listener in times of trouble, but those studies also show that the effects can also cut the other way. Confidants can interfere with the trajectory of a marriage when they take sides, for example, or when they intentionally or unintentionally encourage you to focus on traits in your spouse that irritate or anger you. When your best friend divorces her husband, she may unwittingly push you to more closely examine your own marriage in a way that might make you turn away from it rather than toward it. The Trojan horse is people who care more about your personal, short-term interests than they care about your long-term stake in your marriage.

When Parents Hold on Too Tight

Whatever they thought of your partner when the two of you were courting, most family members get on board once you are engaged.

When the die is cast and the marriage is inevitable, families have a way of embracing the new marriage. In many ways, that's what wedding ceremonies are for, to get everyone on board with the marriage. But sometimes parents are so reluctant to lose their son or daughter to this new spouse that they try to control the couple's lives, thereby creating stress and conflict in the new marriage. (Of course, I am talking about how we handle marriage in mainstream American culture; other cultures would have different expectations and different stresses between newlyweds and their families.)

Take the example of Lonnie and Kate's marriage. Lonnie's mother would have preferred that all of her children live on the same block as she did. She insisted that all major family events occur at her house. She ran Thanksgiving, Christmas, and all birthdays. Kate accepted this deal for several years, until she and Lonnie began to raise their own family. At that point, she wanted to alternate major holidays with her own parents. Lonnie's mother would not hear of it. She told Kate to invite her parents along, but insisted that all gather at her house. It wasn't just holiday rituals, however; it was even Kate's own birthday that had to be celebrated at her in-laws. Lonnie had never stood up to his mother and would not now. Without her husband's support, Kate felt powerless with her mother-in-law and grew resentful of Lonnie for siding with his mother. Lonnie just wanted the two main women in his life to get along.

Lonnie's mother was keeping her son and daughter-in-law from starting their own family traditions based on their own marriage and creating stress between them. Of course, she did not do this alone; Lonnie collaborated by not setting limits on her control, and thus stayed in a loyalty bind between his mother and his wife. To some extent these loyalty binds are inevitable if we love our families and our mate. Different challenges occur at different times in marriage: early on when we shift our priorities to our spouse without abandoning our families; after we become parents when we find a new place for our parents and kin who are invested in our children; and in midlife when we try to balance caring for frail parents with the ongoing needs of our spouse and children. As in any of life's ongoing challenges, a good start helps with the later challenges. Lonnie and Kate did not start out well with his family.

After attending a workshop I did on family rituals, Kate asked to meet with me one time to help her figure out what to do. Together we figured out the following plan of action. She told Lonnie that she wanted his support with his family and that she was going to begin the process of change. She drew her battle line first around her own birthday party, which she insisted, and then doubly insisted, be at her own house. She did not give her mother-in-law a choice. Having won that battle, she then convinced Lonnie to support her on alternating Thanksgivings with her own parents. He agreed to support her. With the couple united now, the mother-in-law had no choice but to begin accepting the limits of her control over her son's marriage and family. It was never going to be an easy relationship with Lonnie's mother, but at least Kate felt better about her marriage.

Nasser and Edie had to settle for a standoff with her parents, but they did keep their marriage together. Edie's parents, from Oklahoma Southern Baptist stock, could not abide her marriage to a Syrian Muslim man. They accused him of using their daughter to obtain U.S. citizenship, and ten years and three children later, they were still encouraging her to divorce him. Although Nasser and Edie did not live in the same state as her parents, this hostility put a lot of stress on her and their marriage. In the early years, Nasser made things worse by continually putting down Edie's family in conversations with Edie, which led to her defending her parents. She did not want to give up her relationship with her parents or her husband. Eventually, after seeking marital therapy to save their marriage, some new realizations dawned on them. Edie and Nasser realized that they could not control her parents' attitudes; they could never make them accept the marriage. Edie realized that she had to grow up and not require her parents' approval in the same way she did as a younger woman. For his part, Nasser came to understand that his criticism stemmed from his own feelings of competition with Edie's parents. Reassured of her commitment, he started to let go of his insecurity. He knew he had to stop criticizing his in-laws because this created a loyalty struggle for her and paralyzed her in setting limits on them.

For the most part, Edie and Nasser stopped arguing about her parents, which helped them keep her parents out of their relationship. Edie insisted that her parents receive her husband into their home on certain family visits, but mostly Edie and the children visited on their own. Their cross-cultural marriage was not without strains, but they did form a united front for the sake of their marriage and their children.

Unless loyalty issues between spouse and parents are dealt with early in a marriage, parents and other family members can undercut a marriage for the long haul. Spouses get into unresolved disputes over whose family is more important and start to begrudge time with each other's families. Some spouses stop visiting in-laws except on major occasions. The underlying issues here are loyalty to the marriage versus loyalty to one's family of origin, and competition between spouses over these priorities. All couples have to grapple with these issues. Here I am highlighting how family members can become underminers of a marriage by pressing, in unfair ways, for their demands for time, attention, and loyalty. When that occurs, you have to fight for your marriage or you will lose it to your extended family.

The key person in the struggle to keep both the marriage and the extended family is the spouse whose relatives are the problem. The in-law can only be a supportive member of the cast, not the lead actor. When I coach people on this process, I often recommend that they decide on their basic, minimum expectations of their relatives toward the spouse and the marriage. For example, the spouse is invited to all extended family events, no unsolicited criticism of the spouse, and no discussions about whether you should have gotten married. You tell your relatives the ground rules, and when they violate them, you can use the "broken record" technique, which involves calmly repeating, over and over until they stop, what you expect. For example, "Mom, you know that I will only come to the party if Martha is invited," or "Criticism of Jacob's religion is off limits."

Almost all relatives will give up the fight if you set limits and calmly enforce them. If they continue to violate the limits, then you can write them a letter and say you are staying away for a time because of their actions. Then call again and ask whether they are ready to resume contact under the ground rules you have set. Remember, though, that your ground rules have to be the basic minimum of respectful behavior toward your marriage, and not a change of heart on your family's part. When they behave respectfully, you can be free to enjoy your relatives, flaws and all, because you are not letting them harm your marriage.

IS YOUR FAMILY OF ORIGIN HURTING YOUR MARRIAGE?

Parents and other family members hurt your marriage only if you let them. Here are some questions to help you determine whether this is happening. Answering "yes" to more than two of these questions might mean that there is a problem. Answering "yes" to more than four means you should take a serious look at where your adult loyalties lie. Answering "yes" to eight or more means you'd better find out if your old room at your parents' house—or your spouse's room at his or her parents' house—is still available.

1. Is the subject of many of your arguments, or your most difficult arguments, how the in-laws treat you or the number of demands they put on your lives?
2. Do you find yourself keeping secrets from your spouse about conversations you've had with your family?
3. Do you find yourself blaming your spouse's minor faults on his or her parents' poor childrearing practices?
4. Does one of you complain that the amount of attention paid to, or time spent with, your respective families is unequal?
5. Do you find yourself trying to preempt invitations from in-laws by making plans with your own parents for holidays and other events without consulting your spouse?
6. Do you feel pressured to agree to plans with your own family without checking first with your mate?
7. Do you find it very difficult to say no to requests from your parents?
8. Do you find it easy to say no to requests from your spouse's parents?
9. Do you celebrate all holidays and special occasions at either your parents' or your spouse's parents' home?
10. Do you feel as if your spouse never sets limits on his or her parents' demands, even when it's clear that they are unreasonable?

If you are concerned about your responses to some of these questions, here are some things you can do to protect your marriage and still maintain loving contact with both of your families.

- If you are in an argument with your spouse about one of your families, avoid retaliating with an attack on the other's family.
- Try not to say anything critical of your in-laws' personalities or family traits that your spouse has not already mentioned. Don't be an eager critic of your in-laws, or you will stir up defensive loyalty in your mate.
- The blood (or adoptive) relative should generally take the lead in setting limits on his or her family. Don't make your spouse the bad guy with your family, and don't become the bad guy with your in-laws.
- If you complain about feeling controlled by your in-laws, there's a good chance the problem is that your spouse is being wimpy with them. Assert yourself with your spouse and insist that your spouse do the same with your in-laws.
- If you feel caught in the middle between your spouse and your family, get out of the middle by seeking an understanding with your spouse, and then having a united front with your family. Staying in the middle means being disloyal to your spouse. Battle it out first with your spouse until you reach a solution you both can live with. When you are setting limits on parents who are expecting too much or acting unfairly, concentrate on stating what you want or expect, over and over if necessary, and stay away from why their entire approach is "wrong."

When Ex-Spouses Undermine

When you have children by a previous marriage, your ex-spouse is automatically a player in your new marriage. If you are fortunate, your ex accepts the situation, or at least is neutral about it. If you are less fortunate, a threatened ex-spouse can threaten your marriage, sometimes intentionally. I have seen ex-spouses sabotage by harassing the new stepfamily. One man called his ex-wife a dozen times a day to complain about the financial and child custody settlement. She would try to calm him down and assert the fairness of the settlement. The emotional toll on her was high, and her new husband complained that she seemed focused on her previous marriage because she spent all her emotional energy there. While guilty, his wife found she was also upset that her new husband was not more supportive.

In our therapy sessions, I helped this couple see that they were allowing the ex-husband invade their marriage. The wife would have to do something she had never successfully accomplished with her ex when they were married: set a limit on his controlling behavior. With her new husband's support, she decided to refrain from answering the telephone at home until she knew from the answering machine whether it was her ex-husband calling. (Nowadays she could use caller ID.) She wrote him a letter stating that she would only communicate via letters for the time being (now it would be e-mail), until he learned to be more respectful. Her new husband felt encouraged by this boundary setting with her ex and became more supportive of her. After a few days of nasty voice-mail messages, the ex-husband ceased intruding. He did refuse to write letters, but he left only necessary voice mail messages about the children's schedules. They were not out of the woods with this man, but at least he was not threatening the new marriage.

Remarriage often means that you have to change your way of relating to your ex-spouse for the good of your new relationship. During your single-parent phase, perhaps you let your ex-husband renege on his weekends with the children because you preferred to have the children with you. Or maybe you had never learned how to deal with his irresponsibility and felt it wasn't worth the argument when he called to cancel at the last minute. But now that you are remarried, your marriage will be hurt if you allow your ex to manipulate you in this way. Your new husband will be looking forward to weekends without his stepchildren, when you can be alone as a couple, and will be angry because he thinks that your ex-husband is jerking both of you around. If you respond by saying that you "feel caught in the middle" between your new husband and your ex, you will make the problem worse. Why? Because "in the middle" suggests that you have equal loyalty to both parties. Instead, you will have to bite the bullet and hold your ex-husband accountable for taking the children when he has agreed to. When he calls on Wednesday to say that he can't take the children for the weekend, you have to say, "Well, I guess you will have to find someone to take them." (This assumes that he has someone competent to care for them.) Otherwise, your ex will determine when you and your new husband can be alone as a couple and will undermine your marriage.

Sometimes the undermining comes from being too close to an ex-spouse. After a year or so of acrimony, Marv and his ex-wife, Ruth, settled into a cooperative, amiable relationship of coparenting with their children. They were exemplary ex-spouses, making decisions well and trading off times with the children as schedules changed. Eventually, Ruth started to share with Marv her personal worries and stresses during their daily phone calls about the children's schedules. This solidified their working partnership, until Marv remarried six years later. His new wife, Barbara, had been aware that Ruth called frequently, but when the new couple moved in together, Barbara was appalled to learn that Ruth called nightly after 10:00 P.M. and that Marv talked with her for a half hour or more. It was clear to Barbara that only the first few minutes were about the children, and she believed that Ruth was deliberately calling at times when she knew Marv and Barbara were free.

Marv, for his part, could not understand why Barbara was upset. Marv was a great listener, a trait that had attracted Barbara to him, but this seemed to Barbara like misplaced compassion. He had no romantic interest in Ruth, he claimed, but he felt sorry for Ruth, who had not remarried and needed someone to talk with about her worries. And he feared that alienating her might compromise their cooperative coparenting relationship. In our counseling sessions, Marv came to see that Barbara had a legitimate complaint about the time and energy he was putting into his personal relationship with his ex-wife, and he decided to make two changes: to talk to Ruth at an earlier hour in the evening, to begin focusing the conversations more on child issues, and to gradually reduce the amount of time spent on Ruth's personal concerns. Barbara felt relieved by his willingness to protect their new marriage from the intrusion of a too-close relationship with his ex-wife.

If you are remarried, how you manage your relationship with your ex-spouse is crucial to the success of your second marriage. Too much negativity or too much positivity can be threatening. Being a warrior toward your ex drains emotional energy from your marriage, as does being a victim. Allowing yourself to be manipulated means that your new mate will feel manipulated—and angry at you. And being too chummy with your ex can make your new mate wonder whether you have really changed canoes.

"Don't Be Tied Down to a Marriage"

At least Lonnie's mother accepted the reality of her son's marriage; she just wanted to control the marriage. Sometimes single friends of a newly married person have trouble accepting the fact that their friend is now in a different stage of life. They encourage their friend to frequent the old singles' haunts on a "night out." I have seen this particularly among couples who marry young, say, in their late teens or early twenties. The issue is not having single friends, but participating in singles' activities with them, such as dancing and bar hopping. One of the spouses sees nothing wrong with accepting these invitations to a singles' bar, arguing with the skeptical mate that it's just for fun, not for pick-ups. The friends love this arrangement because they don't "lose" their single friend, but the marriage usually suffers from jealousy by one spouse and defensiveness from the other, and sometimes from a threatening outside involvement with another person. In most cases I have known, whether it's a "boys' night out" or a "girls' night out," it's a way not to be really married. Single friends can be the first to encourage this dangerous path, and the last to urge its ending. Why? Not because they intentionally want to hurt the marriage (although that might be happening unconsciously), but because they want to hold on to their individual friend through their familiar rituals. But they are not friends of the marriage.

Close friends, including single friends, are an important part of life. But your close friends are either supporters of your marriage or underminers of it. There is no neutral ground. It's the same with parenting; either friends support the importance of your role as a parent, or they do not. They either accept the idea that your marriage relationship is your top priority, or they act as if it is not your top priority. You tell your friend that you've always wanted to go to Hawaii, but that your new husband nixed the idea because he hates Hawaii. Your friend blurts out, "Well, go yourself, then!" The context is that you and your husband each have just two weeks of vacation for your first vacation together of your new marriage. Your friend is supporting your individual entitlement to vacation where you want to, and to not be bossed around by your spouse, but is no friend of your budding marriage.

We have talked so far about family and friends encouraging you to act as if you are not loyal to your mate but to them or to yourself. This kind of undermining can occur in the absence of problems in your marriage, and is mostly likely to occur in the early years of a marriage, when family and friends have trouble accepting the reality of your new commitment. Next we will look at what can happen when you talk to someone close to you about strains and difficulties in your marriage. You are giving another person the opportunity to support both you and your marriage, or only you.

A Friend in Need

I think of Tina, who has experienced her share of personal and marital struggles after marrying young and having two children in quick succession while also attending college. Most of her close friends are still single, and not in committed relationships. Tina is the kind of person who talks openly and frequently about what is causing her stress. She loves her husband, Mark, and is committed to her marriage, but complains that he does not understand her moods and is not supportive enough. When Mark gets frustrated with her complaints about school, for instance, he sometimes ends the conversation by saying, "Why don't you quit school then?"—a comment that she takes as unsupportive of her finishing her education. Although he is a very involved father with their young boys, Tina still carries the majority of the load of parenting and housework. Mark supports the family with a good job.

Mark and Tina sound like many married couples with the stresses that come from having young children and the addition of the stress of having a spouse in college. Their complaints sound like those of many women about their husbands—not enough empathy and not enough work around the house and with the kids. (Mark had his complaints about Tina, but he kept them to himself among his friends.)

Tina, as I said, was quite open with her friends about her marriage. She was looking for support in these conversations, but not for the kind of support she was receiving. You see, nearly all of her friends were fellow college students, and single. After listening to her story, they shared the following kinds of remarks:

> "You deserve better than this."
> "He's completely out of line, and I wouldn't stand for it."
> "I wouldn't put up with a husband like that."
> "Are you really happy in your marriage?"
> "I feel sorry for you."
> "You are such a bright, loving person. I don't understand why he doesn't treat you better."
> "Why are you still there?"

It's the double edge of these comments that makes them so threatening to a marriage. On the one hand, they are so supportive, so affirming of Tina as an individual. Her friends see her point of view, empathize with her feelings of distress, and encourage her to stand up for herself. All good, right? But the other side is that these comments undercut her marriage. Her friends assume that only Tina's side of the story is valid. They don't challenge her about her own behavior. They don't seek to understand what might be going on with Mark. They treat her as the victim in the marriage. And (I hope your ear picked this up), they sing the song of consumer marriage—you deserve more, you are entitled to more, you must be happy at all costs.

Would there be circumstances in which the friends' comments would be fully appropriate? If she were complaining about Mark being abusive or unfaithful or irresponsible with alcohol or money, the friends' one-sided reactions would have made more sense. But the friends' standards were such that most marriages, at some point in their history, would be stressed enough to qualify for these kinds of undermining statements.

Here's another example. A professional woman in a highly committed marriage told me that when she vents her frustrations about her husband's criticisms of her for not being affectionate enough, her friends often say something like, "Why are you still in this marriage?" She has stopped talking to her friends about her marriage.

These kinds of responses from friends would be more appropriate for a relationship other than a marriage, say, a relationship with an employer. "You deserve better. . . . Why are you still there . . . ? I wouldn't stay. . . ." Those lines fit a business relationship in which Tina has not made a vow to love and honor through better and worse until death. It is precisely that vow, and the commitment it represents, that is missing in the comments that friends sometimes make about a marriage in distress.

Colleen told me of her frustrations about how so many of her friends responded to her marital crisis a few years back. She and her husband were struggling with the tumultuous teen years of their son, who had been adopted at age five after an abusive early childhood. Colleen and her husband had vehement disagreements about how to manage their son and about who should be more responsible for monitoring him. Each blamed the other for not being an effective enough parent, although they both knew in their hearts that their son came with many emotional handicaps. This stress, along with their demanding careers, put their twenty-five-year marriage on the edge for the first time. When Colleen opened up to her friends about the problems, she received a consistent message: "The important thing is that you have to take care of yourself." This made her angry because no one was challenging her to look at her own contributions to the problems ("Maybe," she told me, "I was too focused on taking care of myself."). And no one seemed to be advocating for her long-term marriage.

Some friends, on the other hand, support both you and your marriage. They listen to your grievances about your spouse, empathize with your pain, but do not suggest, without obvious good reasons, that your spouse has fatal flaws, that you are getting a raw deal in the marriage, or that you should be reconsidering whether to stay married. There is an art to listening to marital complaints without adding fuel to the fire or taking sides. Friends can ask you, for example, how your spouse might be feeling about the situation. Compassionate friends can also remind you, at the right moment, of what is good about your spouse or your marriage. Being a friend to a marriage is an important but ignored ability in adult life.

A colleague told me about how one of her friends, who also knew her husband well, made a comment that helped enormously during a very dark time in the marriage, when my colleague was actively considering a divorce. The comment was, "I know this is a very hard time for you, and that you may decide to leave your husband, but I want to remind you of something very important: he does love you very deeply." This comment, from someone who loved my colleague, her husband, and their marriage, turned my colleague around in an instant. Many years later, she remains grateful that she did not follow the path of divorce at a time when so many of her own friends took that path.

What kinds of friends are most likely to support you as a separate individual but not as a married person? Never-married friends may not understand the normal stresses of marriage and thereby take your complaints as signs of serious pathology. Never having made a lifelong commitment, they also may not understand it. (Of course, many never-marrieds have a good handle on what is involved and can support your marriage.) Separated and divorced friends may have a stake in your ending your marriage, because it validates their decision to get out of their own marriage and because it means that you become more available as a friend. (Of course, many separated and divorced people want you to avoid losing your marriage.) And family members, if you are in a full-blown marital crisis, might rally around you and demonize your spouse. Unless your mate is truly acting like a demon, this stance undercuts your marriage.

A generation ago we lived in a culture where others would have encouraged you to stay with a spouse who beat you or drank away the family's money. We now live in a culture where more people will encourage you to look to your own needs first and to take a hike if your partner is causing you psychological stress. Fortunately, there are people who will support you as an individual and as a spouse. But you can't always tell who are the supporters and who are the underminers until you invite them into your emotional world. Later in the book I'll describe a new project I've started to help assure that more married people have people in their lives that will support their marriage.

What can you do to resist those who would hurt your marriage if they get inside?

• Choose carefully whom you talk to about your marital problems. Tina, the young married woman with two small children, made the mistake of opening up to too many friends, some of whom did not understand or appreciate marital commitment. People who know and like both you and your mate are more likely to support your marriage and less likely to add fuel to the fire.

• Go to someone who is known for empathy, common sense, and maybe above all, a sense of humor.

• Talk to someone who understands your own flaws well and is not afraid to point out your contributions to your marital concerns.

• When talking about your marriage with family and friends, make sure you balance positives and negatives. Avoid mentioning your marriage only when you are complaining. This may give others the message that you are more unhappy than you are.

• Tell others what kind of support you need. If you want to vent about your mate, tell them that you just need to talk and that you will probably feel better about the situation tomorrow. If you are not looking for advice, say so.

• If your complaints are serious, or you think the other person may see them as more serious than you do, tell the other person up front that you want to make your marriage last and that you are not considering ending it.

• If the other person says something that feels undermining, say that this was not helpful. For example, "Challenging me about why I stay with George is not helpful to me right now because I have already made the decision to work this out. What I need is your support for fixing my marriage." It takes courage to say something like this, and a good friend to hear this. I suggest picking a calm moment some time after the conversation that concerned you, and begin by saying how much you appreciate your friend's interest and support so that she won't get defensive and instead will listen.

Resisting the Call for Low Expectations

There is one more insidious way that family and friends unintentionally weaken our marriages. It's by sending the message of low expectations for married life. This is a variation on the consumer culture of marriage, like saying that the marital lifestyle does not deliver on its promises, so you'd better accept your fate and make yourself happy in other ways. I remember a friend, newly married and very happy, telling me what her sisters and sisters-in-law told her: "It's great until you have kids, and then it goes downhill. But you will always have your kids." These women were not planning to exit their marriages. They saw themselves as realists, and wanted my friend to prepare herself for what was to come.

In a locker room, I once overheard an experienced married man talking to a newly married man. The older man asked what it was like to be married. The reply was "Super." The experienced husband then said something to this effect: "It's great at the beginning, but it changes. For the first time in your life, you can have sex whenever you want it. But after a while, the thrill wears off and you don't even have sex that often." Thus the voice of resignation about sex in marriage.

A related kind of talk among female friends takes the form of mutual husband-bashing, which may, at the time, feel comforting but in the long run can feed into overall negativity. One wife told me that when she or her best friend expressed irritation about their husband, their mantra went like this: "Men are jerks. So what did your jerk do now?" At one level, it seemed like playful banter. But I asked the wife how she would feel if she complained about her teenage daughter and heard back something like this: "Teen girls are self-absorbed brats. What did your brat do now?" A very different response, no doubt. I helped my client see that this kind of banter eroded her respect for her husband even as it might have seemingly built closeness with her friend. Just as putting down a colleague at work might make you feel superior, this kind of spouse bashing (and believe me, it can go the other way when guys talk about their wives whining about dropping everything to watch the game) leads you to feel entitled to something better.

I have two final reflections about this kind of talk about marriage. First, many people take for granted the advantages of being married and then only talk about the downside. For example, loads of research demonstrates that married people have better sex lives than people who are single or divorced. And second, the people who say fatalistic things about marriage have often stopped working on the marriage years ago. Any airplane, any automobile, or any boat can be kept in fine working order for an indefinite period if it is maintained routinely and restored from time to time. Not just the exceptionally well-built vehicles, but virtually every one that functioned well in its early years can be maintained forever. It's the same with marriages, but many people don't know it.

The antidote to the soft undermining of low expectations is to keep in mind that almost everything about marriage can get better as the years go by. Your emotional intimacy can get stronger. Your sexual relationship can get deeper, more varied, and more pleasurable, even if less frequent as you get older. Your ability to have fun together can grow as you relax into accepting each other better. Your joy in raising wonderful children into adulthood can surpass that from any joint work experience in your lifetime. Your roots in a community can be deeper and stronger because they spread out from both of you.

The challenge in dealing with all kinds of messages from others about your marriage is to hold your course while understanding that others will take their own course. Most negative things that can be said about a marriage are true for most marriages some of the time, and for some marriages all of the time. But that doesn't mean that we have to focus on what our good-enough marriage is not giving us. There is insidious power in the "look out for yourself" messages that we sometimes get from loved ones who themselves are influenced by the consumer ethic. That's why having a thriving marriage that is committed, intentional, and community-based is a bold cultural statement in contemporary America.

6 Resist Therapists Who Threaten Your Marriage

If you talk to a typical therapist in the United States about problems in your marriage, especially if you go alone to therapy, you risk harming your marriage. Later on I discuss what you can do about this: how to choose a good therapist and how to get away from a bad one. Here I describe the problem of how some therapists have embraced the consumer culture of marriage and threaten the marriages they treat. I also discuss the sheer lack of training even among therapists who treat couples and how this affects the quality of counseling you can expect if you land in the wrong office.

Keep in mind that I am an enthusiastic couple therapist. I train therapists. I believe that therapy for married people can be very helpful when it comes from therapists who are committed to excellence in its practice, as opposed to those who are mainly individual therapists who dabble in marriage counseling, and who lean toward preserving marriages when possible, as opposed to being neutral about whether a marriage ends in divorce. I first started to talk about this issue in my 1995 book, *Soul Searching,* and I have been growing more concerned since. I am not concerned just about couple therapy, but also about individual therapy, which is where most people talk about their marital problems as part of their life difficulties. I begin with a story.

Paul and Marsha's Near Miss

Soon after her wedding, Marsha felt something was terribly wrong with her marriage. She and her husband, Paul, had moved across the country following a big church wedding in their hometown. Marsha was obsessed with fears that she had made a big mistake in marrying Paul. She focused on Paul's ambivalence about the Christian faith, his avoidance of personal topics of communication, and his tendency to criticize her when she expressed her worries and fears. Marsha sought help at the university student-counseling center where she and Paul were graduate students. The counselor worked with her alone for a few sessions and then invited Paul in for marital therapy. Paul, who was frustrated and angry about how distant and fretful Marsha had become, was a reluctant participant in the counseling.

In addition to the marital problems, Marsha was suffering from clinical depression: she couldn't sleep or concentrate, she felt sad all the time, and she felt like a failure. Medication began to relieve some of these symptoms, but she was still upset about the state of her marriage. After a highly charged session with this distressed wife and angry, reluctant husband, the counselor met with Marsha separately the next week. She told Marsha that she would not recover fully from her depression until she started to "trust her feelings" about the marriage. Following is how Marsha later recounted the conversation with the counselor:

Marsha: What do you mean, trust my feelings?

Counselor: You know you are not happy in your marriage.

Marsha: Yes, that's true.

Counselor: Perhaps you need a separation to figure out whether you really want this marriage.

Marsha: But I love Paul and I am committed to him.

Counselor: The choice is yours, but I doubt that you will begin to feel better until you start to trust your feelings and pay attention to your unhappiness.

Marsha: Are you saying I should get a divorce?

Counselor: I'm just urging you to trust your feelings of unhappiness, and maybe a separation would help you sort things out.

A stunned Marsha decided not to return to that counselor, a decision the counselor no doubt perceived as reflecting Marsha's unwillingness to take responsibility for her own happiness.

It gets worse: Marsha talked to her priest during this crisis. The priest urged her to wait to see whether her depression was causing the marital problem or whether the marital problem was causing the depression—a prudent bit of advice. But a few minutes later, the priest said that, if it turned out that the marital problems were causing the depression, he would help Marsha get an annulment. Marsha was even more stunned than she had been by the therapist. The rest of the story is that they did find a good marital therapist who helped them straighten out their marriage. Marsha's depression lifted, and they are currently doing well, although Marsha knows that she may have to deal with depression on and off throughout her life. They survived two efforts at what I call "therapist-induced marital suicide."

Now, Paul was a very nice guy. But he was young, and he didn't know much about feelings. I didn't know about feelings at his age either, and he was just really befuddled that his new bride was depressed all the time. I had been to their wedding six months before this and was appalled at this turn of events in therapy. How did we get here? It's not that therapists or pastoral counselors are out to hurt people and deliberately undermine marriage. What is going on here?

Where We Have Come from and Where We Are Now

I want to give you my version of a historical overview of the problem I have identified. It was in the 1950s that people really began to pay attention for the first time, in a systematic way, to marital problems. The field of marriage counseling got started then. As we look back at the 1950s from a current perspective, we see a focus on traditional marriage, with traditional gender roles, a reluctance to allow women to be in the workforce. We see divorce being viewed as a personal failing. If you remember, in those days a woman was a divorcée her entire life. If she was in an auto accident, the newspaper headline said, "Divorcée in Auto Accident." A tremendous amount of social stigma was attached to divorce. Therapists often saw divorce as a treatment failure, based on personality problems of an individual. As we look back we often see that the therapist supported certain gender arrangements that society revisited later on. And in the 1950s most people who were doing any work in the marriage area were oblivious to marital violence; it was only in the 1970s that we began to pay attention to that problem.

So what we do in our country is, of course, swing from one kind of model to another. When the 1960s and 1970s came along, we had the rise of the culture of individualism, of marriage based not on duty anymore, but on personal happiness. The dark side of marriage now became apparent as we began to understand the amount of abuse that went on. The divorce rate skyrocketed, no-fault divorce laws began to be passed in the early 1970s, and we had the cultural revolution in which we were liberating individuals from the traditional strictures of conventional morality.

Much of this cultural revolution was an effort to make needed changes. Blinders about the dark side of marital commitment had to be taken away. Older forms of marriage had been based on inequality between men and women, a situation that feminism brought to light. Divorce was so stigmatized that many necessary divorces did not occur. Too many women had been expected to stay in abusive and demeaning marriages. The demand for individual rights in marriage had to accompany the demand for individual rights in the law and workforce. But as in most other cultural revolutions, there were many unfortunate side effects that we must now struggle with.

Therapists took two stances toward marriage during the 1970s. The first stance was "neutrality" on the subject of marital commitment. In a short time, therapists moved from an era in which a prominent psychiatrist in the 1950s said that he never supported a couple's decision to get a divorce, to an era where the therapist was supposed to be neutral. A survey of clinical members of the American Association for Marriage and Family Therapy found that nearly two-thirds said that they are "neutral" on the subject of marriage and divorce. A poll in Minnesota asked divorced people about their experience with marriage counseling. Only thirty-five percent of divorced people believed that their therapist wanted to help save their marriage, forty-one percent believed the therapist was neutral on whether the marriage survived, and fourteen percent said that the therapist encouraged the divorce. I mentioned earlier what a prominent family therapist told the press a few years ago, "The good marriage, the good divorce, it matters not." Is this what you are looking for when you seek help for your marriage, or when your son or daughter seeks help?

The other stance emerging during the 1970s was beyond neutrality, to therapists seeing themselves as liberators to help people out of unhappy marriages and other commitments in their lives. We had the introduction of the idea of liberation from marriage, particularly when somebody sees an individual therapist. If you describe your marriage as painful for you, the therapist wants to liberate you from this toxic influence. This stance is still with us. If someone raises a concern about the fate of their children, many of us were trained to say that kids will do fine if their parents do what they need to do for themselves. That's what I used to say at the beginning of my career.

As we talked about earlier, the 1980s and 1990s were a time when market values—the norms of the marketplace—triumphed in American culture. Consumerism prevailed. If the 1970s were the "I gotta take care of my own psychological needs" decade, the 1980s added the element of material greed. The business model invaded everywhere. As I've said, I'm not against the business model in business, but look how it has invaded the professions, with healthcare facilities talking about "guest relations" and universities having "customers" (previously known as "students"). It should not be surprising that therapists began to see consumer marriage as the norm and to treat married people as self-interested parties in a "limited partnership."

How Therapists Undermine Marital Commitment

I believe that there is a lot of unnecessary pain and unnecessary divorce created by incompetent therapists and by therapists who take hyperindividualistic approaches to marriage. In this view of marriage, marriage is a venue for personal fulfillment stripped of ethical obligations. And divorce is a strictly private, self-interested choice, with no important stakeholders other than the individual adult client. The result is, in my opinion, that it is dangerous in America today to talk about your marriage problems with therapists unless you know what their attitude is and what their skill level is.

Now I'm going to talk about the most common ways that therapists undermine marital commitment. And I want to underline again that I believe in therapy. I do this for a living. I think that therapy can be enormously helpful in the right hands. I see four main ways that therapists undermine marital commitment: through incompetence, through neutrality, through seeing only marital pathology, and through active undermining of marital commitment.

• *First, incompetent therapists.* The biggest problem I see in this area is that most therapists are not trained to work with couples, and they see working with couples as an extension of individual psychotherapy. It is not. In individual therapy, depending on your model, you can be laid back. You can be empathetic and clarifying, you can even be fairly passive if you want, and be very helpful to individuals in therapy. People will tell their story, they will feel heard, and they will think through their concerns and their options. As experienced marital therapists know, and as the research on marital therapy indicates, if therapists take a laid-back approach in marital therapy, they will fail. If you have a warring couple in your office, and you do not create a structure for that session, they will overwhelm you. They will repeat in the office what they do at home. A lot of therapists end a stormy session with, "Well, we've clarified some of the issues, haven't we?" Which means they've put in psychological terms the stuff that the couple already knew they were doing. And these therapists offer no direction, no structure, and no guidelines—under the pretense that this is being helpful. This may be helpful to some individuals in therapy, but it is not helpful to couples.

WHAT TO LOOK FOR IN YOUR THERAPIST: DOS AND DON'TS FOR A COMPETENT MARITAL THERAPIST

Most people don't know what to expect of a competent marital therapist. Here are some qualities and actions that researchers have found to promote effective marital therapy.

Dos

1. The therapist is caring and compassionate to both of you.

2. The therapist actively tries to help your marriage and communicates hope that you solve your marital problems. This goes beyond just clarifying your problems.

3. The therapist is active in structuring the session.

4. The therapist offers reasonable and helpful perspectives to help you understand the sources of your problems.

5. The therapist challenges each of you about your contributions to the problems and about your capacity to make individual changes to resolve the problems.

6. The therapist offers specific strategies for changing your relationship, and coaches you on how to use them.

7. The therapist is alert to individual matters such as depression, alcoholism, and medical illness that might be influencing your marital problems.

8. The therapist is alert to the problem of physical abuse and assesses whether there is danger to one of the spouses.

Don'ts

1. The therapist does not take sides.

2. The therapist does not permit you and your spouse to interrupt each other, talk over each other, or speak for the other person.

3. The therapist does not let you and your spouse engage in repeated angry exchanges during the session.

4. Although the therapist may explore how your family-of-origin backgrounds influence your problems, the focus is on how to deal with your current problems rather than just on insight into how you developed these problems.

5. The therapist does not assume that there are certain ways that men and women should behave according to their gender in marriage.

Another thing that incompetent therapists do is focus on only one partner's problems and turn marital therapy into individual therapy, with one spouse off the hook. In couple work, this sometimes occurs when the therapist can't handle the in-session conflict and feels overwhelmed by it. This work is not easy. The pulls, the triangles, the hot conflict right in the room make this therapy very challenging for the therapist. The problem isn't just that some therapists can't handle it. The problem is they don't know they can't handle it, and they assume that there is a lot of individual psychopathology in one or both spouses. They stop helping the couple because they think that one or both spouses must do individual therapy before they can work on their marriage. Meanwhile, the marriage is hanging in the balance. I have seen a lot of unnecessary divorces because of this scenario.

• *Second, neutral therapists.* In the 1970s and 1980s, I was a neutral therapist on marriage and divorce. I helped people do a cost–benefit analysis—what the individual gains and loses by staying married or getting divorced. This consumerist cost–benefit analysis disguises itself as neutral. A sole emphasis on the questions "What do you need to do for you?" and "What's in it for you to stay, what's in it for you to not stay?" are not neutral because they focus only on what the individual sees as his or her own personal gain or loss. Neutrality when somebody has previously promised before their family and community, and perhaps before their God, to be married to this person until death parts them—neutrality on whether somebody can fulfill this commitment—is an undermining stance, not a neutral stance.

Neutrality often means siding with the more self-oriented spouse even when the partner wants to work to save the marriage. A common stance among couple therapists is to refrain from offering hope for the marriage when the spouses differ on whether to try therapy. I call these "mixed-agenda" couples—one leaning toward divorce and reluctant to do therapy, and the other wanting to save the marriage. They are the bane of couple therapy because therapists often do not know how to work with people who have different goals. I will talk more on this later when I discuss in greater detail how to find the right therapist. For now, it's important to know that when the neutral therapist offers little hope for the marriage, the result is an alliance between the reluctant, distancing spouse and the therapist, a collusion that undermines the marital relationship in ways that the therapist probably does not recognize.

As an alternative to holding a neutral position, I let couples know that, except in situations that are either abusive or dangerous, I will support the chance that the couple can salvage their marriage. I see myself as an advocate for their marriage. They can call me off, but they're going to have to look me in the eye and call me off. I'm going to try to support the possibility they can work this out, knowing that they too must want it and that it is not always possible. Other therapists might say this differently, but they will communicate the idea that salvaging your marriage is their first priority unless there are clear reasons to take another course.

• *Third, therapists who see only pathology.* This is really an insidious one. You go to individual therapy, you criticize your spouse, and your therapist comes up with a psychiatric diagnosis for your spouse: "I'm afraid you're married to a narcissistic personality disorder." When you get a therapist giving you labels to pathologize your partner, it leads to hopelessness. Sometimes the therapist pathologizes the reason you got married. For almost any marriage, therapists can figure out what pathology fed its inception. This can lead to a sense of fatalism and hopelessness. You should never have bought that car to begin with; it was a lemon from the get-go.

Another version is to pathologize the current relationship, telling the individual or couple that they have no marital assets, that this is a sick relationship, and that anyone who stays is in questionable psychological health. Let's say you see an individual therapist after your spouse has an affair, and you're thinking of taking your spouse back. You may be pathologized for your very commitment to keep trying. What's wrong with you that you are hanging in there? The therapist can highlight a one-sided sense of victimization. Or take the introduction of the word "abuse" to describe ordinary marital conflict. There is a lot of genuine physical and psychological marital abuse out there, and a competent therapist will assess your marriage for abuse (including talking to each of you individually about this when appropriate). But the term "abuse" gets thrown around a lot. You can take ordinary unhappiness and conflict and transform them into the sense of being abused. You were unhappy, took and gave back a goodly amount of negativity, but now your therapist has convinced you that you are a victim of your spouse, and this then propels you out of the marriage.

A final form of pathology is one for this era of turboconsumerism: being "bored" with one's marriage. I've seen therapists get very exercised about how awful it would be to be in a boring marriage and be quite sympathetic to why these spouses have affairs and move on to new partners. In a consumer culture, when we want stimulation and satisfaction all the time, boring is the new marital pathology.

• *Fourth, overt undermining.* A common way that therapists hurt marriages is through provocative questions and challenges. "If you are not happy, why do you stay?" is a directly undermining question. It suggests, "You are an idiot if you stay, because your main goal in life is to be happy." I had a student who had postpartum depressions after both of her children. She went to counselors to get help, in the process complaining about her husband for being insensitive to her emotional distress, but never saying that she was doubting her commitment to the marriage. Each time, at the end of the first session, the therapist made some version of this statement: "I can't believe you're still married to him." This is an assertion of the therapist's belief that the couple are fundamentally incompatible, that she is entitled to more, and that an intelligent client should run, not walk, out of the marriage. You'd be amazed at how many therapists say this kind of thing after a session or two. Without knowing it, what they are often saying is not that the couple are fundamentally incompatible but rather that "I am fundamentally unable to help you." Of course, this plays into the agenda of the distancing spouse who is considering divorce.

Then there is undermining by direct advice. It's against the code of ethics of most psychotherapy organizations to directly tell people what they should do, either to stay married or to get divorced, but a lot of therapists do it anyway through direct advice to take care of oneself. They don't say, "I think you should break up," but they say, "I think you may need a separation," or "For your own health you need to move out." In one case, a woman with a husband and ten children relapsed from her alcoholism. Her individual therapist told her that she needed to move out and have minimal contact with her husband or kids, for the sake of her recovery. The family therapist I talked to was trying to pick up the pieces with the husband and children, who could not understand why their mother's "recovery" meant this kind of cutoff.

Monica and Rob Dodge a Therapist's Bullet

I'd like to tell you another story, this one happening to a couple I knew personally. This was the story that propelled me to become an activist, to sound an alarm.

Monica was stunned when Rob, her husband of eighteen years, announced that he was having an affair with her best friend and wanted an "open marriage." When Monica declined this invitation, Rob came unraveled emotionally and bolted from the house. He spent the next week in a mental hospital for an acute, psychotic depression, and was released to outpatient treatment. Although he claimed during his hospitalization that he wanted a divorce, his therapist had the good sense to urge him not to make any major decisions until he was feeling better. Meanwhile, Monica was beside herself with grief, fear, and anger. She had two young children at home, a demanding job, and was struggling with a serious chronic illness she had been diagnosed with twelve months ago. Indeed, Rob had never been able to cope with her diagnosis, or with his own job loss six months afterward. (He was now working again.)

Clearly, this couple had been through huge stresses in the past year, including relocation to a different city where they had no support systems in place. Rob was acting in a completely uncharacteristic way for a former straight-arrow man with strong religious and moral values. Monica was depressed, agitated, and confused. She sought recommendations to find the best psychotherapist available in her city. He turned out to be a highly regarded clinical psychologist. Rob was continuing in individual outpatient psychotherapy while living alone in an apartment. He still wanted a divorce.

As Monica later recounted the story to me, after two sessions of assessment and crisis intervention her therapist suggested that she pursue the divorce that Rob said he wanted. She resisted, pointing out that this was a long-term marriage with young children, and that she was hoping that the real Rob would reemerge from his midlife crisis. She suspected that the affair with her friend would be short lived (which it was). She was angry and terribly hurt, she said, but determined not to give up on an eighteen-year marriage after only six weeks of hell. The therapist, according to Monica, interpreted her resistance to "moving on with her life" as stemming from her inability to "grieve" the end of her marriage. He then connected this inability to grieve to the unresolved loss of her mother when Monica was a small child. Monica's difficulty in letting go of a failed marriage, he insisted, stemmed from unfinished mourning from the death of her mother. I call this an attempt at therapist-induced marital suicide.

Fortunately, Monica had the strength to fire the therapist.

Not many clients would be able to do that, especially in the face of such expert pathologizing of their moral commitment. And equally fortunately, she and Rob found a good marital therapist who saw them through their crisis and onward to a recovered and ultimately healthier marriage.

How to Find a Therapist Who Will Support Your Marriage

Therapists don't advertise that they routinely undermine marital commitment, and in fact no ethical therapist would see himself or herself that way. Many therapists genuinely believe that individual well-being should be their own concern. As one local therapist likes to say to clients, "I'm not here to save marriages; I'm here to help people." How do you avoid seeing a therapist who separates the good of individuals and the good of marriages? And how can you find someone who is likely to be competent as well as supportive of your marital commitment? Here are some questions you can ask on the phone.

• "Can you tell me about your background and training in marital therapy?" If the therapist is self-taught or workshop trained and can't point to a significant education in this work, then consider going elsewhere.
• "What percentage of your practice is marital therapy?" Avoid therapists who mostly do individual therapy, because they are not likely to be skilled in working with couples.
• "Of the couples you treat, what percentage would you say work out enough of their problems to stay married with a reasonable amount of satisfaction with the relationship?" "What percentage break up while they are seeing you?" "What percentage do not improve?" If someone says "one hundred percent" stay together, I would be concerned, because some marriages should end. If therapists report less than seventy percent stay together and work out their problems, then their success rate is below average (based on

studies of the effectiveness of marital therapy). And if they say that staying together is not a measure of success for them, I would not see them for therapy because they are in the camp that is neutral about marital commitment.

- "How do you see the importance of keeping a marriage together when there are problems?" If the therapist responds only with the language of consumer self-interest ("I just try to help both parties decide what they need to do for themselves"), then follow up with a question about whether the therapist holds any personal values about the importance of marital commitment. If the therapist just repeats the mantra of people doing what they have to do for themselves, then go elsewhere if your values differ.

To help people find therapists with pro-commitment values, I joined with my therapist daughter Elizabeth Doherty Thomas to create a values statement. If you agree with this values statement, you might want to keep it in mind as you talk with a prospective therapist. If you want to be more assertive, you could read or mail the statement to a therapist before you make the first appointment, or show it to the therapist at the first appointment. You could couch your query with something like the following: "In a book I read about marriage, I came across a list of values about how therapists should help married couples make decisions about staying married or getting divorced. I liked the list, and I wonder if you would be willing to look at it and let me know how you feel about it."

I recognize that this could be a delicate discussion because you might fear coming across as confrontational with someone you want to trust. But I think it's worth it if you don't know from a third party what the therapist's stance is. And if you are a professional who refers couples to therapy, you could use the statement as a way to screen for therapists who share your values. I wouldn't focus on whether every therapist would agree with every word or phrase, but for the general level of agreement or discomfort with the gist of the values statement.

Before giving you the values statement, I want to take a moment to comment again on the good side of consumerism, the side that emphasizes that individuals have a right to full knowledge about what goods and services they are purchasing. Any therapist who seems critical of your politely worded questions, or who is reluctant to disclose his or her beliefs about marital commitment, is not treating you with respect as a consumer. You should look elsewhere.

VALUES STATEMENT
(www.takebackyourmarriage.com)

1. Because healthy marriage is a source of human flourishing for individuals, families, and communities, I affirm the unique value of marriage as a lifelong commitment.

2. Because most troubled marriages can be restored to health if both partners apply themselves vigorously to make that happen, my first stance as a therapist is to help them preserve their marriage and find a path to a better relationship.

3. Because love and fairness must go hand in hand, I promote the needs and goals of both partners.

4. Because marriages have other stakeholders, especially children, I help couples see how others are affected by the success or failure of their marriage.

5. Because some marriages become hazardous to health and well-being, I do not promote marital commitment blindly but rather with respect for safety and human dignity.

6. Because people have the ultimate responsibility to make their own decisions about staying married or divorcing, I respect these decisions even if they differ from what I hope for the couple.

7. Because the stakes are often high when marriages are in distress, I seek consultation when I feel stuck in therapy or when the couple is moving toward what may be an unnecessary or premature divorce.

The Cultural Tide Is Shifting

I see the culture shifting again, as we reconsider the fruits of the consumer culture. We're moving toward what I believe is a better balance between individual satisfaction and moral commitment, and toward the creation of new opportunities for people to learn how to have lifelong, successful marriages. But I believe that many therapists are behind the times. Like generals, therapists are still fighting the last war, the one that freed individuals to leave unhappy marriages. Many of us still see ourselves as liberation fighters for individual fulfillment against oppressive moral codes and family structures. That's how I started my career as a therapist.

But in the meantime the culture has changed. The old war has been largely won. Most of us are now free to walk away from our marital commitments more easily than from any other contract in our lives. We can always get a divorce if "things don't work out," and we suffer relatively little social stigma for doing so. But now we face the prospect of losing our ability to sustain any commitment at all. We have cut through our marital chains but ended up with Velcro. Easy to pull apart, but not strong enough to hold us together under pressure.

Speaking of pressure, I think of long-term marriage like I think about living in my home state of Minnesota, in Lake Wobegon, perhaps. You move into marriage in the springtime of hope, but eventually arrive at the Minnesota winter with its cold and darkness. Many of us are tempted to give up and move south at this point. We go to a therapist for help. Some therapists don't know how to help us cope with winter, and we get frostbite in their care. Other therapists tell us that we are being personally victimized by winter, that we deserve better, that winter will never end, and that if we are true to ourselves we will leave our marriage and head south. The problem, of course, is that our next marriage will enter its own winter at some point. Do we just keep moving on, or do we make our stand now—with this person, in this season? That's the moral, existential question we face when our marriage is in trouble.

A good therapist, a brave therapist, will help us to cling together as a couple, warming each other against the cold of winter, and to seek out whatever sunlight is still available while we wrestle with our pain and disillusionment. A good therapist, a brave therapist, will be the last one in the room to give up on our marriage, not the first one, knowing that the next springtime in Minnesota can be all the more glorious for the winter that we endured together.

7 Preventing Unnecessary Divorce

Until now, we have been focusing on forces that pull couples apart in our modern world: the natural drift of intimate relationships, the consumer culture, children who own us, time that gets away from us, and family and friends who take sides. Here I want to talk about how to take back your marriage when these and other forces have gotten the best of you and are moving you toward an unnecessary divorce. Then the rest of the chapters in this book will lay out ways to build, or rebuild, your marriage.

I like to distinguish between "hard" and "soft" reasons for divorce. Hard reasons are problems such as the three "A's": abuse, addictions, and affairs. These problems undermine the possibility of safety and trust in a marriage. Their degree of seriousness is measured by their pervasiveness in the relationship. Is the affair ongoing and the spouse unwilling to end it? Will the offending spouse take responsibility for her actions, like the spouse who won't seek help for her addictive behaviors or a partner who demeans, belittles, and emotionally abuses and insists it's all your fault?

Studies have shown that within the past generation we have moved from divorcing for mostly hard reasons to divorcing for softer reasons like communication problems and lack of intimacy. Along with my colleagues Alan Hawkins and Brian Willoughby, I recently gave a standard checklist of reasons for divorce to nearly nine hundred divorcing people with minor children.

The two reasons given by more than half of divorcing people

were growing apart and not being able to talk together. The next five most frequently cited were how the spouse handles money (forty percent), infidelity and personal problems of my spouse (thirty-seven percent), not getting enough attention (thirty-four percent), and the spouse's personal habits (twenty-nine percent). Alcohol or drug problems made the top ten at twenty-two percent. These findings, which are similar to those found by other researchers, show that most divorces are not based on severe problems that compromise health and well-being, but on more subtle relationship problems that might be more easily repaired. This is not to say that lack of intimacy and personal connection, the hallmarks of today's divorces, are not deeply painful. And I am not suggesting that most people walk away from their marriages for superficial reasons. But both the research and my clinical experience suggest that with early intervention and hard work many divorces could be prevented without compromising the health and safety of the spouses.

I'm going to focus here on preventing divorce for the soft reasons, but I want to say something about the hard reasons. Nearly any serious personal problem someone brings to a marriage is treatable if that person owns up to the problem, seeks proper help along with the spouse, and dedicates himself or herself to becoming healthy again. This is true in many cases of affairs, addictions, and even some violence when the abusive party is firmly committed to change. (Couple therapy researcher Constance Stites has shown that many couples with a history of violence can be effectively treated.) Of course, there are spouses who are entrenched in their behavior, do not take responsibility for change, and in fact blame their mate for the problems in the marriage. In those cases, the other partner may have no choice but to leave. But absent dangerous situations, I encourage people who are considering leaving for hard reasons to take some time to learn about their participation in the unhealthy relationship. Some clients, for example, did not set limits on unacceptable behavior, or assumed responsibility for dysfunctional spouses. For example, attending Al-Anon meetings can shift the experience of wives who have lost their bearings in an alcoholic marriage. By moving in a healthy direction before you call it quits on the marriage offers two benefits: it gives the marriage the best chance to survive and it helps to avoid the same mistakes in future relationships if your current marriage ends.

In my own practice with spouses (usually women) who still love their husband and would stay married if he changed, I help them deliver a complex and challenging message to their mate: "I love you and hope that we can save our marriage. But I can't stay married to you as long as you are doing. . . . I know that I have changes to make if we are going to have a good marriage in the future, but right now I am saying that I can't keep working on our marriage unless you take what I am saying seriously and commit to changing." (You have to know what you are asking for: not just promises but action— for example, getting a substance abuse assessment, going back to AA, ending an affair, or starting couple therapy.) One wife said it this way to her husband about his denial of his drinking problem: "Unless you deal with your drinking problem, you will have me as a housemate but not a wife." That was his wake-up call for starting treatment and finally getting healthy again.

There are two main paths that couples take toward unnecessary divorce for the soft reasons, and you need to know how to avoid those paths and get off them if you find yourself there. The first path is the slow way of small choices that eventually bring down a marriage. The second path is the fast track. In either case, with wisdom, courage, and support, you have a good shot at turning your marriage around. An unnecessary divorce is one of the great tragedies of adult life, and all roads toward it are agonizing.

Small Choices, Big Losses

You can bring down almost any good marriage in two years. You start with focusing on what you are not getting out of the relationship and how your partner fails to live up to your expectations. Below is a game plan you can follow; I have seen it work many times.

The sad part is that the one who initiates it does not realize, until it feels too late, that this is a marital failure path. It's a slow, steady path without markers that say "Stop; Turn Around." I will frame the story from the wife's point of view, because women initiate two-thirds of divorces, but with some modifications it could be a husband's story as well. It's a composite of many couples I have worked with.

Your husband is not particularly good at supporting you emotionally. He loves you, is a good father, and is rarely mean to you, but doesn't know what to do with you when you are emotionally upset about something in your life. He doesn't listen long enough, or he tries to fix your feelings by giving you unwelcome advice. Maybe he gets exasperated after a while and suggests that you should stop worrying so much. In other words, he acts like lots of men who were never raised to have long, empathetic, give-and-take conversations.

At some point in the marriage, you begin to focus more on your husband's deficiencies as a supportive confidant. Why now? Maybe you are more stressed these days, or you are aware of a gradual drifting apart emotionally in your marriage, or you realize that a good friend's husband does a better job. A dangerous reason is that you have a new male friend who really listens to you but whom you do not talk to your husband about. Being a secret confidant over a latte is far easier than being an open confidant in a full-time relationship that comes with a house and kids. Or maybe you've reconnected via the Web with an old flame; it starts out like a fun friendship but by not telling your husband, you risk becoming emotionally attached in a way that could threaten your marriage.

Whatever the reason you are especially bothered right now, it's probably not because your husband has changed stripes. He never was particularly adept at the kind of supportive listening and responsiveness that you would like. And you married him anyway, because he has lots of other good qualities, and you have been pretty happy together. If there is a gradual decline in emotional closeness in your marriage, especially after the kids came, you are probably as responsible for it as your husband is.

For whatever reason, you now begin to obsess about what you are missing because of your husband's deficiencies. Aren't you entitled to more support? Isn't it appalling that he can't give you what you need and deserve? Why is it that you can talk to your friends but not to your very own husband? Don't you do a far better job of supporting him? The books you are reading about marriage point to something much better. It's completely unfair! How can you be expected to live this way? You have to change him.

The next step can take two different paths. First, begin to criticize him for how he responds to you; tell him he doesn't know how to communicate, and that he thinks only of himself. This will likely elicit defensiveness and counterattack from your husband, which will prove that he is an emotional dolt and not willing or able to "be there" for you emotionally. Marital researchers such as John Gottman have documented how these negative conflict patterns propel couples toward divorce. (For advice on effective problem-solving skills in marriage, see his book *The Seven Principles for Making Marriage Work*, and Howard Markman, Scott Stanley, and Susan Blumberg's book *Fighting for Your Marriage, Second Edition*.)

If you have these battles often enough, over a long enough period of time, you or your husband might start to use the "d" word (divorce) in your fights. You bring it up, or he does, to get the other's attention, not because either of you really means it. But the possibility of divorce has now entered your communication for the first time. Even if it's not on the table, it slithers and hisses around on the floor like a snake no one wants to notice.

You can take a second path from the start, or after failing at the first path. Here you withdraw from your marriage by not sharing your feelings about anything important. Chances are, your husband will think that you are not troubled about anything these days, and will not notice, for a time at least, that you are not being open. You withdraw sexually, without giving a reason—which your husband certainly notices. You enter an emotional shell. After marinating there for a while, you will see yourself as the victim of an empty marriage that is cutting off your emotional air supply. You do not notice that you had a big role in putting yourself in the shell.

Having begun two years ago with a common and nonfatal problem with your marriage, you are now at the point of deciding to separate and divorce. The internal emotional logic at this time is compelling: you are living either in a high-conflict, stressful marriage or in a lonely, empty marriage (or maybe cycling through the two). You are now convinced that you and your husband have become different people and have irrevocably grown apart. You're sure that he'll never change or your relationship improve. You get support from your friends and maybe a therapist (here they are again), who agree that you are miserable and need to move on.

As you process the history of your failed marriage, you now believe that it was fatally flawed from the beginning. The two of you were not right for each other; you were on a rebound from another relationship; he did not have the capacity to grow that you did, and so on. (Divorce researchers have demonstrated how we revise our stories about the history of the marriage to fit our current desire to end it.) Your husband by now is not talking to you anymore—or shouting when he does talk—and is as clueless as you are about how to save the marriage. He is still hoping that things will work, but you are not.

Research on the divorce process shows that before announcing the divorce, you will likely make an escape plan. You have checked out your financial situation and your housing needs. You have consulted with divorced friends, who, along with your therapist, support your conviction that your marriage is beyond repair. You read books about how to do divorce well, and tell yourself that as long as you and your ex-husband remain friendly as coparents, the children will come out okay. You may be actively fantasizing about better romantic partners, and you may be turning to one for platonic support—or more. When you finally drop the bomb on your husband, he is shocked. He says he didn't see it coming, and you are amazed. You agree to go to marriage counseling, but your heart is not in it. You are relieved that the therapist concurs that your marriage cannot be saved. People in your life who see it otherwise either don't understand or are laying a guilt trip on you. You have embarked on the divorce phase of a journey you started unwittingly a year or two before. If you are lucky, you will not repeat the scenario in your next marriage, but chances are good that you will, especially under the stress of stepchildren. Second divorces come much more quickly, on average, than first divorces, especially when we haven't learned from the first one.

Notice how the wife (as I said, it could be a husband too) focused nearly exclusively on her husband's deficiencies, not on her own. This is the consumer mind-set: my marital needs are not being met, so there must be a problem with your marital performance. I see more people nowadays whose only admission of responsibility for marriage problems is that they chose the wrong person, or maybe put up with that person's failings for too long. If my car does not perform well, it's not my fault; it's the manufacturer's. Never mind that I drive it too hard and don't change the oil.

How could the wife have handled the situation as an active citizen of her marriage, someone who is responsible for building and repairing the relationship, and not as a consumer of the marital lifestyle? She could have recognized her wish for more empathetic support from her husband as a "desire" and not a core "need." She would then approach the issue with less sense of entitlement and victimization. She could try letting her husband know what kinds of responses she finds helpful, without criticizing him. She could suggest that the two of them take a course in marital communication, so that she could get out of the role of being his coach in marital communication. She could suggest a couple of sessions with a marital therapist to tune up their couple communication.

She could also just accept that emotional empathy is not her husband's strong suit, and may never be. She can ask him to just hold her when she is blue or upset, and then talk through all her feelings with a good friend. Everyone has some needs that do not get met in marriage. This is not tragic unless we make it that way; it is just life. I remember the moment when Susan stopped dragging her husband into therapy every two years to get him to open up with his feelings. During a therapy session, he tearfully told her that he didn't think he was built emotionally the way she wanted him to be, and he was sad that he could not be a better husband for her. Susan understood for the first time that his nonemotional way of living did not reflect on his love for her. And, ironically, this made it easier for him to be a bit more open with his feelings, as he had been in this counseling session.

Harry, another client, had been preoccupied with his wife's lack of interest in sex. He took this very personally and would get angry with her. It's the kind of struggle that can blow up a marriage over time. When it came out in therapy that his wife had been sexually abused as a child, and was having trouble being touched sexually,

Harry successfully worked on accepting her as she was. With the control struggle diminished, and the threat to the marriage taken away, they both relaxed and slowly rebuilt a physical relationship.

Alexis, age fifty-four and married for thirty years, avoided an unnecessary divorce by means of what she called "an attitude adjustment." Her husband, Ron, took early retirement at age fifty-five from his company and decided to just hang out at home, puttering in his hobbies. Alexis kept working. She had expected that Ron would find another job, and found herself increasingly annoyed and disappointed that he "sits on his butt all day." He did pick up more of the housework when she asked him to, but it did not seem right to Alexis that her previously productive husband was a homebody. When she suggested he get a job, he became defensive, pointing out that his pension was bringing in more than his share of the family income. She retorted that they could not afford to live in their current house on their combined income. He agreed, but would not get a job to keep the house, which he claimed was too big for them now anyway, with their kids grown and gone. So they moved to a smaller house, to Alexis's disappointment.

After simmering for more than a year, Alexis had a hard conversation with herself, as she put it. She told herself that she could either continue to work herself up about Ron's lifestyle or she could accept it. Ron was sick of the world of paid work and was not going to return to it. They had enough money to live a middle-class lifestyle. She was working a job she enjoyed and was not ready to retire. Ron had relieved some of her load of housework and household management, and he did projects for their grown kids and their young families. Alexis saw that the heart of her irritation was the idea of an able-bodied man occupying the house all day and not seeking employment, leaving her the only paid worker in the household. But she did not want a divorce and realized that she could be working herself up to one. So she decided to stop feeling so sorry for herself and so frustrated with Ron. She still wished he would get a job and not sit around so much, but with an "attitude adjustment" she started to manage her disappointment with more equanimity and began to enjoy his company again for the first time since he retired.

Alexis and Ron's story is not out of the textbook on marital problem solving, where spouses are taught to air their feelings and wants, and then reach a compromise that works for both of them. Sometimes it goes that way in marriage, but other times one spouse cannot or will not make the changes the other wants or needs. In a culture of personal entitlement and frequent divorce, this is often the moment of decision about beginning the road to divorce or staying off that road. The actual decision to divorce may be years later, but we set ourselves in motion at a much earlier stage. Even if we start that journey, we can decide, like Alexis, to switch paths when we realize where we are heading.

What helped Alexis and many other spouses to avoid an unnecessary divorce was a stark look at where they are headed if they continue on the path of resentment about not getting their needs and expectations met. In other words, they realize that the small choices to emphasize the problems in the marriage are building up to a big decision on whether to stay married or get divorced. An analogy would be what we now know about cancer: a full-blown cancer occurs only at the end of a series of steps that go awry, like a succession of switches that each turn "on" instead of "off." Many divorces come after dozens of small decisions to emphasize the bad and downplay the good about the marriage or the spouse, to avoid looking at one's own flaws and to focus on better options with another mate instead of learning to live better with the mate you have. Again, I am not referring to situations of abuse and chronic infidelity, which should not be tolerated. I am referring to the softer problems that turn hard by how we deal with them. By ratcheting up our own disappointments, we can turn our mate into someone we want to leave. By accepting our mate's limitations, and realizing that our own flaws are usually of the same caliber, we can get on with the work of getting our canoe back upstream.

The Fast Track to an Unnecessary Divorce

Most of my examples have been with established marriages of some duration. With new marriages without kids, unnecessary divorces can take the fast track, and it calls for quick work to pull them back from the cliff. The most vulnerable years of marriage are the first two. Sometimes even before the couple are adjusted to each other, it's over. Here is Mary Sue and Josh's story.

Not long after their honeymoon, Mary Sue is upset that Josh is hanging around too much with his old friends and not spending enough free time with her. He stops by at his favorite bar after work for an hour or so, a habit that inflames her. When she confronts him, he doesn't want to talk about it, except to claim that she is being too possessive. Her friends agree with her completely. His friends say that he is henpecked. They still have a lot of love and good will for each other, but are wondering whether they should have gotten married or continued to live together. They didn't have such bad arguments then. Mary Sue wonders whether she pushed Josh too hard to get married, but he had not wanted to lose her. Both are from divorced families and are nervous about what marital commitment means.

This is a couple in need of a community of friends and supporters to help them adjust to marriage. But like most couples in the land, they are on their own, struggling with what it means to be married and not having particularly good skills for tackling their problems. Shockingly, one day during a fight Josh blurts out, "Maybe we should just get a divorce." Taken aback but angry, Mary Sue retorts, "Maybe we should." Neither of them wants this, but neither of them will take it back. One of Mary Sue's divorced friends later warns her that Josh could be taking all the money out of their bank account, and that she had better protect her interests. So she talks to a divorce lawyer, who starts the legal process and files papers on a stunned Josh. In Ramsey County, Minnesota, where this couple lives, it is possible to get a divorce in one week, from first visit to a lawyer until the final decree, if you do not have children and no one contests the terms. Usually it takes longer because of the court docket, but it has been done within one week. Josh and Mary Sue pack up and move on with their lives, with little understanding of what happened.

Josh and Mary Sue needed time and help to grow into the responsibilities of marriage, but they pulled the trigger of divorce too fast for them to learn together. What they needed was a rapid response from their family and friends, and perhaps their faith community. More mature adults could tell them emphatically that they were faced with growing up and becoming married adults, and that their problems were common—and manageable with time and patience. One immediate step would have been for them to get into marital therapy with a therapist who was willing to support their efforts to mature individually and adapt to being married.

Marsha and Jeff were more mature, but faced an immediate set of crises when Marsha's mother and father died in an accident. She was devastated, and Jeff did not know how to react to her grief and distress. She felt disappointed and abandoned by Jeff. In her despair, she thought that divorce was the only alternative to staying with a man who could not support her. Fortunately, this couple got help from a therapist who supported Marsha and the marriage, and they emerged stronger. The key step was Marsha's realization that Jeff didn't know how to support her. It wasn't that he didn't care. She also realized that she did not have to turn only to Jeff for support; she could lean on her friends too. Her feelings of betrayal melted away, and she could justify staying in the marriage and finding ways to improve it. For his part, Jeff did work on connecting with Marsha, at least not moving away from her when she was upset. Marsha and Jeff were nearly an early casualty of our "return this lemon to the dealer" mentality toward marriage and divorce. Thank goodness they found the right therapist. And how sad that they did not have a larger community to help them through their crisis.

We are getting smarter in this country about helping new parents adjust to having a baby in their midst. There are visiting home nurses and low-cost parent education services available. There are scheduled doctor visits. Families at risk get more intensive services. But for new marriages, we offer little after the big sendoff at the wedding. No one can know whether Josh and Mary Sue could have achieved a long-term marriage, but it is clear that their divorce now was premature and unnecessary because, unlike Marsha and Jeff, they did not seek help and did not give each other more time. Their marriage lasted less than a year.

When There Is Just One "Soft" Problem, but It's a Big One

Sometimes a marriage is good in most ways, there is no abuse, addiction, or affairs, yet one problem can be a marriage breaker. The affected spouse wants desperately to save the marriage but feels that he or she cannot live with the situation. But especially when the marriage is otherwise okay and there are children involved, it's not so clear that leaving is the solution. And yet, staying feels tantamount to being cheated out of something important in life. Here is an exchange of e-mails with a woman in this situation. When you finish reading her letter, I suggest that you pause and reflect on what you would say and on the messages of this book before you go on to read my response.

Dear Dr. Doherty:

I was reading Sunday's USA Weekend and came across an article on divorce in which you were quoted regarding how divorce in a low-conflict marriage is devastating on kids. It quotes you to say that "it is no longer clear to you that when parents leave a non-destructive marriage to pursue your bliss or because you don't want to give children a bad model of marital intimacy." I am really interested in learning more about "enlightened" thinking in this area.

Your description of a non-destructive marriage hit close to home. I have been struggling with what to do for almost three years now and my overwhelming priority is to do what's best for the kids. I've also read your speech on how therapists can be counterproductive to saving marriages and wholeheartedly agree. We went to two therapists and I am disillusioned with therapy and would not recommend it to anyone. Both therapists pretty much gave up and told me to live with the situation (which they doubted I could do for long) or get a divorce. My husband and I get along great day to day for the most part, we are very family centered, consistent and collaborative in raising the kids. To the outside world we appear like a very happy, extremely stable family. The problem is that he says he doesn't love me as a "wife" but cares for me as a person (but has no interest in anyone else), he has no desire to try to save/start-over in a romantic relationship with me but he has no desire and is not willing to voluntarily leave.

I think he would stay with me forever. I'm the one struggling with living this way. Generally I'm happy with my life but it torments me that I'm living a lie. In addition, sleeping in the same bed every night with someone that doesn't even touch you makes me feel so rejected. I don't want to bore you with the whole story but I am looking for some grounding, something to help me put things in perspective, make a decision and make a plan to live with that decision for the long term.

The issue alluded to in the article about the model we are setting for our children is one I have struggled with. I agree that they are not oriented to their parents' sex life but not seeing their parents express any physical affection for each other, isn't that bound to make an impression? I have a son and a daughter. I worry particularly about my son. I want them to have emotionally and physically fulfilling lives.

I suspect you get thousands of e-mails like this and I'm sorry for going on. Just writing has released the stress of the day. Any sources you could refer me to that address the issues I raise from an intellectual and spiritual perspective would be greatly appreciated.

Thanks for your time.

Dear _____,

I am sorry to hear about your painful dilemma, and I don't have any easy answers. To your question about the effect on your kids, a divorce will certainly harm them more than living with two loving parents who do not openly share physical affection. If you become so distressed by the situation that it affects your parenting, that would be the way your children would be harmed by your staying.

For me, it would make a difference if my spouse was psychologically or physically unable to be interested sexually, versus dismissing me and the problem. I would not know which it was until my spouse joined me in a full-court-press effort to get help to change things. I would want my spouse to hurt for me and herself that she could not respond. Then it would be like accepting a spouse's chronic illness. I don't know if your husband has made this kind of effort, or if he has been half-hearted and selfish in saying "I am the way I am." If he has not thrown himself into the effort to make things better, then I might consider insisting on a full and long effort at therapy with a really good physician and a really good therapist, the goals of which would be either restoring your sexual relationship or both of you accepting the sad but painful (to both of you) fact that your husband has a disability in this area. The other thing is that a spouse can be physically affectionate even if he or she cannot respond sexually. If your husband refuses to join you in this effort, then I would be inclined to precipitate a marital crisis—putting the possibility of divorce on the line—not because he can't respond sexually but because he is being irresponsible about a core dimension of the marriage by not being willing to go the extra mile for your sake, for the marriage, and for the family.

If you decide to try this and let me know where you live, perhaps I can help you find a good therapist.

Whatever you decide, I admire you for taking your marital commitment and the needs of your children so seriously in an era where many people would have split long ago.

Bill Doherty

Taking Your Marriage Back from an Unnecessary Divorce

When there is an unnecessary divorce, there has usually been a failure of leadership in the couple. With some couples, neither of them really want the divorce, but neither speak up to stop it. In other cases, spouses either complain frequently about a problem, but do little more than nag or occasionally rage about it. They argue about who is more at fault. No one steps forward to say that the marriage is in trouble, and that they had both better do something to preserve it.

ARE YOU ON THE VERGE OF AN UNNECESSARY DIVORCE?

When divorce leaves the realm of "it couldn't possibly happen to us" and creeps into the domain of "maybe that's what I will have to do," the idea often gains a tragic momentum of its own. Unfortunately, if you've reached this point, the pain and fear you feel may be enough to blur your perception of reality and your judgment about the best course of action for you and your marriage. Some couples don't take the warning signs seriously until it feels too late. If more than three of the following statements describe you, drop everything and make a commitment right now to put off any decision or actions to dissolve your marriage until you get real help.

1. You're beginning to claim that you and your spouse were really never in love, yet your friends and family say you were crazy about each other when you got married.

2. You say your spouse never pays any attention to you and never makes an effort to spend time with you, yet somehow you're busy—with work you brought home, with volunteer meetings, with dinner or a drink with friends, with helping your child with homework—every evening of the week.

3. These days you dwell mostly on your spouse's faults and failings but if pressed to describe the type of person your spouse is, you would use terms like "fair," "dependable," "responsible," and "kind."

4. You say your partner can't be a good spouse, but is a good parent. You rule out the possibility that someone who can be a good parent might also be able to learn to be a good spouse.

5. You begin your usual long litany of complaints about your marriage to your mother or a friend, but for the first time the response is "Maybe you're right to think about divorce," and you find yourself speechless as well as surprised to feel a little hurt.

6. You say you're determined to be "done with it" and get on with your life, but you've canceled appointments for an initial consultation with a divorce lawyer.

7. You make constant declarations that you want to work things out with your husband, but your once-benign fantasies about having an affair are beginning to take shape in reality—a work colleague asks you to lunch, an e-mail correspondent turns flirtatious, or you are pleased that the guy you play tennis with is getting divorced.

8. You say that you crave emotional connection, but when your spouse is unavailable, you watch television instead of calling a friend. You may not be such a great emotional connector yourself.

9. You feel as if you've tried everything and despair that anything will ever get better, even when you know your spouse is trying to change.

10. You know you will have trouble explaining to your children, now and in the future, why you ended the marriage. You are not sure that ending the pain you are in now justifies the pain that they will be in later.

Surveys in the United States and Australia have shown that forty percent or more of divorced people regret their divorce and that the great majority of divorced people believe that one or the other of them could have worked much harder to save the marriage. My own research has found a lot of ambivalence in divorcing couples even up to the time of the divorce decree; in fact, in forty percent of divorces at least one partner thinks the marriage could still be saved. Researchers also tell us that generally there is a "leaver" and a "leavee" (the one left) in a divorce. Rarely are both parties on the same page at the same time. In unnecessary divorces, both may carry the responsibility for lack of leadership. The leaver generally does not openly disclose his or her level of dissatisfaction, in order to not rock the boat and out of a sense that nothing can be changed. The leavee generally prefers to keep his or her head firmly in the sand, for the same reasons. It's hard to live daily in marital crisis, and so, outside of arguments that burst forth occasionally, most of us keep quiet about worries about our marriage. But this means that no one is naming the problem in the marriage and no one is stepping up to the plate for the relationship. Two consumers, no leaders.

Leadership for the marriage is different from fighting for your own needs, although that can be a form of leadership, too. It's fighting for your marriage, for the "us." As my colleague Terry Hargrave expresses it, every marriage has a you, a me, and an us. Most struggles between spouses are over the you and me—who gets their way more, who gets their needs met better. In consumer marriage, advocating for me is what I am supposed to do. Lots of books on marriage focus on this. The idea is that if you advocate for your needs and I advocate for my needs, and if we both are skilled at this communication, all will be well. As I have said before, self-advocacy is important in marriage, but it is not enough. Ultimately, when our canoe hits the sandbar and gets stuck, one of us may have to push harder for the sake of both of us, for the sake of the marriage. This is marital leadership.

In the best marriages, both people are leaders, although sometimes at different times. What I want to convey, though, is that each spouse is personally responsible for finding a way back from the precipice when the marriage is threatened. If your mate is demoralized, as is often the case when the marriage is on the rocks, then step forward yourself to take the initiative. If you wait for a joint initiative, it may never come. If your partner temporarily drops an oar, you have to steer by yourself for a while.

When Monica, the wife whose husband had the affair and wanted a divorce (I discussed them in Chapter 6), faced an emotionally unraveling husband and undermining therapist, she asserted herself and said, "Slow down. I am not leaving this marriage. I will keep the communication lines open with my husband. I will let him know I am terribly hurt but still want to save our marriage. I will not dump all my anger on him right now, because that would not be constructive. I will find a better therapist." This is courageous marital leadership.

Art had messed up his marriage by repeatedly lying to his wife about his use of the family credit card for making pornographic phone calls. He got into individual therapy, and I saw the couple for marital therapy. The issue was deeper than pornography and lying, of course. Angela, his wife, saw these as examples of his long-term irresponsibility in the marriage, where she felt like the only adult. She herself could be volatile in her anger and did not see her contribution to the problems very well. One day, in a rageful moment after an argument, she announced that the marriage was over and that Art was to move out. (They had two school-age children.) I saw them for an emergency therapy session. Calmer now, Angela was still determined to end the marriage. She was tired of the work and saw little promise of change, she said.

Art, for the first time, stepped forward with confidence. He said that he would not move out because he believed their marriage was salvageable, that he was straightening himself out, that the children needed an intact family, and that Angela was making a bad decision that he would not cooperate with. Angela repeated her insistence that Art leave by the end of the week, and he repeated that he would not go but would stay and show her that he could be a responsible, loving husband. (He knew that it would take weeks before Angela could legally get him to leave, since there had been no abuse in the marriage.) A month later, Angela changed her mind. They had moved back from the edge of divorce, in part, because Art exercised leadership for the marriage, perhaps for the first time in their life together. They went on to repair their marriage.

Here are some ways to take a stand for your marriage when it is threatened, either in the early stages of breakdown or in the more threatening stage of near divorce.

• Speak about the good of your marriage, not just about your own good. Instead of just saying, "I need you to listen to me more, and you are not doing it," you can add, "I'm sure that it's hard for you that I am so upset with you about this. This is not good for our marriage."

• Decide you are going to work on personal, unilateral change for the sake of your marriage. Some couples divorce because they get into a standoff about who is going to change first. Should the pursuer stop pursuing first, or should the distancer stop distancing first? Someone has to start, preferably telling the other what you are doing and why, so that they know what is happening. My colleague

Michele Weiner-Davis's book *The Divorce Remedy* is the best guide I have seen to making personal changes to salvage a marriage.

• Ask yourself about whether you are expecting your mate to meet all your needs and whether you can accept the fact that you will have to meet some needs elsewhere. I am not referring here to your need for personal safety and freedom from emotional abuse, but to the long list of personal needs that no one human being can meet for us.

• If you are very angry or frustrated with your spouse over an ongoing problem, ask yourself whether this is a "marriage breaker" if nothing changes. A spouse's repeated affairs might be in that category, or an ongoing chain of hostile and demeaning behavior toward your children in a remarriage. But if, as is most likely the case, the problem is not one that you would leave over, even if it is not resolved, then say so. Let your spouse know that this problem does not shake your commitment to the marriage, but is nevertheless causing you pain and you want to resolve it. The advantages of this kind of clarity are twofold: it clears up any doubt your spouse might have about your intentions, and it may help your spouse not get his or her back against the wall during the argument.

• If your spouse uses the "d" word (divorce) in an argument, say clearly that you do not want to divorce, that you want divorce off the table, and that you will do anything to make your marriage work. Ask for an agreement that neither of you will use that word in an argument because it overwhelms the conversation and can create a momentum of its own.

• Insist that the two of you get help together. This can be in the form of marriage education classes, and retreat experience such as the Retrouvaille program, or marital therapy with a therapist who will support your marriage. Don't accept "no" from your spouse about this. Not seeking help for a failing marriage is a form of irresponsibility akin to not seeking medical attention when a family member is seriously ill. Ultimately, if your mate refuses to go, seek help yourself with someone who will help your marriage and keep inviting your spouse.

• If your spouse asks you to move out, and you want to salvage the marriage and genuinely change yourself to do so, refuse to move.

Say that you are determined to save the marriage and will not cooperate in ending it. But if you have been abusive or your spouse is afraid of you, you should move out when asked and continue to work on the marriage from a distance.

• Even if you are separated, you can keep working on the marriage by working on yourself. Use the separation as a wake-up call to become a better person and the person your marriage needs. I remember a wife who was determined to be a healthier, more assertive person after her husband left; she actually concurred with his complaints about the person she had become. He was amazed by her changes, intrigued by who she was becoming, and moved back in.

To avoid an unnecessary divorce, it is not enough to start with a loving commitment, or even with a religiously grounded commitment. With nearly half of new marriages ending in divorce, many divorces occur to people who start with heartfelt commitment, backed by religious convictions. The battlefields of divorce are strewn with the carcasses of couples who started out with love, commitment, and good intentions. As stresses and dissatisfactions mount, they need marital leadership to stay afloat.

Marital leadership is more important today because the external sources of glue for marriage are no longer as strong. It used to be that social pressure would keep people together long enough to work out their problems, or at least not to leave for the soft reasons without a real effort. (Social pressure kept some destructive marriages together too.) Religions that condemn divorce, or set a very high bar for justifying it, used to provide an external source of glue for troubled couples. In tight-knit communities, the town elders might intervene if a couple showed public signs of distress and instability. Nowadays, therapists are supposed to help but, as we have discussed, cannot necessarily be counted on. And family members and friends are often skittish about intervening into your "privacy."

We've got to change this isolation of couples in crisis, but in the meantime, the leadership to avoid an unnecessary divorce usually must come from within the marriage. It's down to you and your mate to muster all your courage, wisdom, and agility to dodge that lethal bullet and start taking back your marriage. Stopping the steps to divorce is just the beginning of recovery, like retrieving your boat from the rocks. You still have to do the hard work of rowing, which means being committed no matter what and intentional about your ways of connecting, and finding a community of people who care about your marriage. That's where we are heading with the rest of this book.

8 Intentional Marriage
Connection Rituals in Everyday Life

The biggest threat to good marriages is everyday living. That may sound strange to you. What I mean is getting lost in the logistics of everyday life. We spend most of our time at home managing a household, taking care of children, and pursuing solitary activities like watching television or working. Having children especially seems to doom personal time for conversation between spouses, and even the time we do have is dominated by logistical talk about schedules and household tasks. At best we feel like effective co-managers of a family business. At worst, we feel like ships passing in the night. By the time the kids leave home, we may not remember how to be different with each other.

But it doesn't have to be this way. The key to growing a marriage that is personal, and not just logistical, is to be intentional about the connection rituals of everyday life. If more couples did this, I am convinced that a lot of divorce lawyers and marital therapists would be put out of business. Doing it is within the reach of all of us, no matter what our family backgrounds or personal problems or past marital problems.

What Are Marital Rituals?

Rituals are social interactions that are repeated, coordinated, and significant. This is the classical, anthropological definition. Rituals can be everyday interactions, or they could be once a year, but they're repeated. They're also coordinated. You have to know what is expected of you in a ritual; you can't have a meal ritual together if you don't know when to show up for it. You're not going to have much of a sexual life if you don't end up in the same space at the same time. But rituals are not only repeated and coordinated, they are significant. A ritual must have positive emotional meaning to both parties.

This matter of significance is what distinguishes a ritual from a routine. A marriage routine is something that you do over and over in a coordinated way, but that does not have much emotional meaning. You can have dinner together as a couple every night, while one of you watches television and the other is absorbed in an iPad. This is probably a routine because it lacks emotional significance. Of course, one couple's routine might be another's ritual. I have a friend who is very busy, as is her husband (their kids are grown). She told me about the mundane activity she and her husband do every Saturday that helps her feel close to him: they do errands. For them, this is a ritual of connection. You see, if they did their shopping efficiently, they would divide up, right? Rituals are not efficient; they are about connection. So my friend and her husband do errands together and talk along the way.

Now that we've defined a marital ritual, let me distinguish several types. Connection rituals, the focus of our discussion now, are rituals of everyday life in which the spouses share time and attention with each other. They are often low key as opposed to intense, comforting as opposed to sparkling. Connection rituals are at the base of the pyramid of marriage, right above commitment. Two other types of marital rituals are love rituals and special occasion rituals. We will discuss both of them later. Love rituals are more intimate ways of interacting than connection rituals; they are how couples express their deep affection and passion for each other. The major special occasion ritual for marriage is the anniversary, but there are other possibilities as well for couples to mark important times in their lives together.

Rituals of Connection in Marriage

Almost anything can be turned into a ritual of connection, if the focus is on the relationship. Some couples check in with each other by phone a couple of times a day. It's only a ritual, though, if both of them know it's a connection time. If just one person likes to call and the other person says, "Yep, yep, busy, busy, I'll talk to you later," this is not a ritual, because it is not coordinated—and it's probably not emotionally significant either. In fact, the demand–withdrawal cycle ruins rituals; both people have to be into it.

Examples of connection rituals include good-byes in the morning, greetings in the evening, and going out for coffee and conversation. I talked to a woman who said she and her husband always say "I love you" when they part in the morning, because they never know that they will see each other again. Working in the garden together can be a connection ritual. I bash the effects of TV on marriage, but I know a couple who, when they watch a favorite TV show, sometimes take turns giving each other a shoulder rub, with one sitting on the floor and the other on the couch. My wife and I have a couple of favorite TV shows that we relish watching together and analyzing afterward. We feel a common joy when they are renewed for another year. The key is to watch the show as a couple ritual— and then turn the TV off—rather than slouching in front of the tube all night.

As we discuss marital rituals of connection in more detail, I'd like you to think about your own rituals, as I share some rituals from my marriage and from those of others. Remember: To be a ritual it must be repeated, coordinated, and significant to both of you. It can be small or large. Some of them start with what psychologist John Gottman calls "bids," small gestures in words or actions by which one partner reaches out to the other. When the other responds positively, it's a successful bid. When these become part of the fabric of the relationship, they become rituals. Taking your spouse's hand in yours on a walk is an example; it changes an exercise walk into a way of connecting—as long as your spouse holds your hand back!

I start with greeting rituals in my own marriage. I don't remember what Leah's and my greeting ritual was before we had kids. But I do know it degenerated at some point. This might be our greeting at the end of the day: Leah to Bill: "Hi. Eric threw up, and Beth has been obnoxious." Bill to Leah: "The garage door is on its last legs." Thus the greetings from the love of one's life! Many of us greet our coworkers more personally and with more enthusiasm. Leah and I realized that this greeting routine was not working for us anymore, and we decided to try something different by intentionally saying: "Hi, honey. How are you?" with a hug and kiss. Pretty radical, huh? Like people who are in love. You heard it here first, and I've taken out a patent on it. You'll have to pay us fifty cents every time you do it.

I once asked a couple I was seeing in therapy about their greeting ritual. Karen was usually home first and working in the kitchen. The four children and the golden retriever were somewhere else in the house. This is what would happen: The husband, Ron, walks in, greeted first by the dog with a big, enthusiastic show of affection. Dogs are great ritualists. They are consistent, they are loving, and they are excited to see you. You can actually chart the number of hours you've been gone, and correlate that with the energy of their greeting ritual. So Ron walks in the door, is greeted by the golden retriever, and next by the kids, with hugs all around for children numbers one, two, three, and four. And then he goes to the bedroom and changes clothes. Karen remains in the kitchen. Some time over the next twenty minutes Ron wanders into the kitchen and the first words uttered by one or the other are something like, "Jesse has a concert tonight, so we have to hurry up dinner."

I asked Karen and Ron how they had greeted each other when they were newlyweds. With sheepish grins, they recounted that it was "Hi, honey, how are you?" followed by huggy, kissy, and "How was your day?" I asked them if they remembered when that had changed. They couldn't even guess. Most of us are clueless about the decline in our marital rituals. Rituals erode just as gradually as the Mississippi wears at the shoreline.

And so I asked Karen and Ron whether they wanted to continue with their current greeting or to change it. We spent an entire session working on the first sixty seconds after Ron came home. Why do I suggest such careful deliberations, like working out land sharing in a peace accord? A greeting ritual is like a choreographed dance that will only work with both people answering the following questions in the same way: Who approaches whom first when they meet? How do they want to actually greet each other? With physical contact? Is the physical contact a hug? A kiss? If a kiss, on the lips or on the cheek? This degree of intentionality in restoring the ritual is important. Otherwise, the scene will go like this: In he walks, expecting her to find him. Meanwhile, she's expecting him to find her. No greeting occurs, and resentment builds if they had set out to change their greeting ritual. You have to decide who takes the first step in the dance. Remember: rituals are coordinated.

Karen thought that a hug and a kiss on the cheek was all she was ready for. I affirmed her honesty here. Otherwise, the first time Ron tried to kiss her on the lips, she would pull away. And he would say to himself, "What the heck is this about, anyway? I am trying to be affectionate and she rejects me." And then he won't approach her again.

In the intricate rituals of married life, both God and the devil are in the details. Which is why the crafting of good marital rituals requires care and thoughtfulness. With some help, Karen and Ron restored a simple greeting ritual as a way to learn to be intentional in their marriage and to reweave, thread by thread, the fabric of their relationship. It started with him finding her in the kitchen when he came home. They exchanged a hug and a kiss on the cheek, and asked each other about how their day went. Nothing fancy, but it helped them feel like a married couple again.

I did a workshop once for couples in which I talked about greeting rituals and asked for participants' own examples. One of the participants said that she and her husband, like Karen and Ron, have a golden retriever and kids. A while back, the couple had noted their dog's consistently high levels of enthusiasm for greetings, and they decided to create a greeting ritual to top their golden retriever. Top the dog, they decided. After all, they were not married to the dog. So now what they do is rush toward each other, jumping in the air and waving their arms, squealing with delight like this: "Wooo! Woooo!" I had them demonstrate. This couple decided to go over the top in their greeting ritual. And they did it every day. Now this is a one-of-a-kind ritual that would never have appeared on my top ten list. But it is so wonderfully playful. And what do you think it's like for their children to watch this? Our children note how we greet each other, whether with the golden retriever maneuver or just a simple hug, kiss, and expression of gladness to be reunited with our mate.

The Special Case of Talk Rituals

Let's now talk about talk rituals, which are an important type of everyday connection ritual. Every marital advice book stresses the importance of taking time to communicate. But if a couple with children has fifteen minutes of uninterrupted, nonlogistical, nonproblem-solving talk every day, I would put them in the top five percent of all married couples in the land. It's an extraordinary achievement. When I say that to college students, they can't believe it. When we are courting and falling in love we have oodles of time to talk. More than sex, it's talk that propels most of us to fall in love and want to get married. After we get married, or if we live together but don't have kids, we still have time to talk, but even then our time is starting to erode because of the TV, the Internet, cellphone, and general household management. If we then have kids, time to talk takes a big dive. You're not going to have time for personal talk, if you have children, unless you ritualize it. Mumbling at eleven o'clock at night when you are exhausted does not count as a talk ritual.

Earlier I mentioned a talk ritual that Leah and I came up with when our youngest child was four. After dinner, we would clean up, give the kids dessert, start the coffee, and then send the children off to play. We taught them to leave us in peace while we had our coffee, so that we could talk. We asked them to not interrupt us unless the house is burning or something equivalent, in which case they can always call 911 and then interrupt us. This ritual gave us about fifteen minutes every day to talk as a couple.

Phases of Marital Rituals

Our daily talk ritual has the three phases involved in all rituals. First, a clear transition. Anthropologists refer to this as the transition to ritual space. It simply doesn't work to say, "Let's just find fifteen minutes every evening." If you don't specify a time, then someone initiates it at an inconvenient time for the other, say, when one of you is doing the laundry or finishing e-mails. Even if you do specify a time but don't anchor it to a transition point in the schedule (like at breakfast, after dinner, or at bedtime), one of the spouses has to track down his partner to remind her that it's time to connect. After doing this for a while, he or she says, "Hey, I'm always reminding you that it's 8:30 and time for us to talk. How come you don't start our talk ritual?"

It works better to have a clear, regular transition point that is calibrated to some event. For us, the time was dinner, followed by coffee. Of course, if one of us has to leave immediately after dinner, we do not have the talk rituals, but we always note the exception. One of the ways you know you have a solid ritual is that, when you cannot do it for some reason, you mention that fact. If you just skip the ritual without commenting, you communicate that it is not important.

The first phase of a ritual, then, is the transition to ritual space. The second is the enactment phase, when you are actually engaged in the ritual activity, in this case a conversation. Here Leah and I evolved the following ground rules: no logistics talk, such as who paid the gas bill; no problem-solving talk, such as what are we going to do about the leaking gutters on the house; and no conflict talk, such as "Now that I've got your attention, let me tell you how upset I am about what you said to me last night." If you do logistical talk, you will not connect at a personal level, so why do the ritual? If you do too much problem-solving talk, it's like work. And if you let conflict enter the conversation, then one or both of you is likely to start avoiding the talk ritual because you may not feel up to working so hard on your relationship.

In fact, avoiding unnecessary conflict is an important ground rule for all marital and family rituals. (Almost all conflict issues can wait until later.) If you go out on a date, do not bring up unpleasant topics. Do not discuss your problems when the goal is to enjoy each other's company. As adults, we are fully capable of opting not to raise irritations and grievances. We visit annoying relatives all the time and avoid squabbles, right? We can decide to be pleasant with our mate for fifteen minutes a day, or on a date, without heroic effort. But we have to be intentional about it.

What Leah and I actually do during our talk ritual is an emotional check-in. It's "How are you doing?" "What has your day been like?" It's just a check-in. No problem solving, no logistics—just being friends savoring a brief interlude of personal conversation every day of their married lives.

The third phase of a ritual, after the transition and the enactment, is the exit stage. You have to have a clear, coordinated way to end the ritual. The problem with saying, "Well, we'll talk for a while" is the ambiguity about when it should end. Somebody may be just warmed up when the other is looking at the clock and winding down. You get into a pursuer–distancer pattern if you don't know when the ritual ends. If you're out at a restaurant, the exit phase usually is clear because the waiter gives you the check. With our coffee ritual, it generally takes about fifteen minutes to drink a full mug of coffee; when our cups are empty, we more or less are ready to stop. This is a clear exit signal, with no need to negotiate. Negotiating every time is inconsistent with ritual, because there is too much opportunity for struggle, which undermines ritual.

Rituals morph over time. When the children left home and my schedule involved more evening meetings, our reliable connection time shifted. As you know, it gets cold in Minnesota, so we bought a hot tub and put it outdoors under the stars. Our nightly ritual of connection, begun some twenty-five years ago, is that around 10:00 P.M., we go to the hot tub. We sit under the stars and talk. Again, no logistics talk. And every time we've fallen into the trap of discussing a conflict it has not been pretty.

I only understood how the hot tub had become a marital connection, and not just an individual pleasure ritual, when Leah started traveling more. I realized that when Leah is out of town, I didn't use the hot tub very often; it's a couple thing. A struggle over the hot tub ritual taught me another lesson about what it means to us. At one point, yours truly, Mr. Ritual Expert, began to say, "I don't think I feel like doing our hot tub talk tonight." After a few times of this, Leah expressed concern that we were losing something that was good for us. We had a discussion about what this meant, with me taking the individual rights approach, the authenticity approach, the consumer approach, if you will. I said, "Are we talking about a rule here? Suppose I don't really feel like doing the hot tub?" I came to realize in that discussion that the hot tub was a couple ritual that was good for "us," even if I was not interested in it for me. We don't do the hot tub if we've been out late or there is thunder and lightning or a blizzard. But otherwise and for the most part, we do our hot tub ritual. It's been part of our marriage for many years.

I will mention a final talk ritual. A client couple were very disconnected, low in conflict but disconnected. The wife would get home from work around 8:30 at night, and usually they did not talk much during the rest of the evening. But they came up with the following talk ritual. When she came home, he would find her and greet her. He would start the water for tea while she changed clothes. And then she would go to the living room, he would bring in the tea, and they would sit and talk. Can you see why the details of this ritual are so important? There was a clear transition mark: she comes home, he greets her, and then he starts the water. For the enactment, they had an agreed-upon place to talk, a place without many distractions. (They had a teenage daughter who was happy to leave them alone after her mother visited with her for a few minutes.) The exit phase began when they finished their tea.

This nightly connection ritual was a way back in to feeling like a married couple. But you only know you have a real marital ritual when you lose it, and then put it back. Rituals are always threatened by erosion, like the shores of the Mississippi. This couple went on vacation, during which the tea ritual was not practical. When they returned home, they failed to put the ritual back in place, and then they realized they missed it—and reinstated their tea time. You always lose a ritual for a time, and then you have to decide how important it is to you.

The Creativity of Couples' Connection Rituals

When I do workshops on couple rituals, I always ask for rituals couples have created on their own. I am always stunned and inspired with the creativity that comes forth. Some couples write regular love letters to each other. In one long-term marriage, they have a closet full of them—and the kids are going to read them when the parents are gone. Some couples shower together every night and snuggle in bed to warm up. Many couples, including me and Leah, end every day in bed with an "I love you"—without fail, and no matter how tense the evening has been.

Some connection rituals are brief verbal exchanges that have meaning only to the couple. When people share them with others, they are sometimes a bit embarrassed at the silliness, but these exchanges serve as small rituals that make the couple unique in the world. One couple make animal sounds to each other. Another have this exchange every night before going to sleep: After they turn out the lights, the husband makes his way across the bed in the dark and embraces her, whereupon she says, "How do you know it's me?" And he answers, "Nobody else would ask such a stupid question!"

EVERYDAY WAYS TO TAKE BACK YOUR MARRIAGE

- Establish a set time every day to talk—just to check in, with no discussion of money, children, or chores.
- Create a greeting ritual that marks the moment and has meaning for the two of you.
- If you've stopped going to bed together regularly, start again.
- Leave an affectionate note for your spouse that has no practical purpose.
- Start dating again. Go out on a spontaneous date or plan one right now.
- Spend more quiet time together without the TV on.
- Move the TV out of your bedroom.
- Notice something you like about your spouse and share it.
- Take one small step tomorrow toward the marriage you would like to have this time next year.

Maybe aside from the daily love letters, none of these rituals takes extraordinary effort. Couples mostly evolve them by happenstance, and then continued to do them intentionally and with commitment. Our rituals define us as couples.

If at this point you are feeling bad because you don't have many good connection rituals in your marriage, then I encourage you to remind yourself about other areas of strength in your marriage. No marriage tops the charts in every area. If you want to beef up your marriage with better connection rituals, share your interest with your mate. In Chapter 12 I share strategies for putting rituals into place in your marriage and sprucing up the ones you have. In the meantime, let's move on from connection rituals, the bread and butter of marriage, to love rituals, the spice.

9 Intentional Marriage
Love Rituals

People from cultures with arranged marriages think that our "love marriage" system is odd. From their perspective, we entrust this highly important decision to young people who are in the throes of infatuation instead of to wiser adults who can be more objective. This said, while I would never want to return to arranged marriages, we do have something to learn from an observation made by advocates of arranged marriage: if marriage is like a pot of water in our system, the pot is at its hottest at the beginning of the marriage and progressively cools over time; in their system, the water starts out cold and is expected to increasingly heat up. But our way of marriage does not have to result in lifelong cooling, if we practice love rituals all of our years.

Here is a love ritual of a couple married more than thirty years and with four children. At random times during the year, Gary buys his wife, Cathy, a rose and hides it somewhere in the house. The rose is always a different color. He never tells her where he has placed it, allowing her to be surprised and delighted when she comes upon it. She sees it as his "I love you" message.

I call these love rituals because their main purpose is to say "I love you and you are special to me." The rose ritual comes with no words, but both know what the meaning is. Other love rituals involve the words themselves. When Laura and Ryan see each other during the day, one might say, "Honey, did I tell you how much I love you today?" and the other will reply, "I don't think so."

As I read these words, I am struck by how schmaltzy they look in print. Love rituals are not meant for outsiders' ears, but it can stimulate our imaginations to hear them anyway. Luke and Marianne have a love ritual on long car rides when, at least several times each trip, one will notice the turn of a new hour and say, "It's a new hour. Have I told you how much I love you lately?"

If you are like me, you may be feeling a bit inadequate right now. When my wife and I are on a long car ride and a new hour passes, I am more likely to say, "I'm falling asleep at the wheel" than, "Have I told you lately how much I love you?" One couple's love ritual opportunity is another's "let's keep on trucking." The point is not that we imitate one another's specific ways of saying "I love you," but that we understand the power and potential of love rituals in our marriage.

Okay, so what do Leah and I do for love rituals? For one thing, after we married we never gave up dating. Not when our children were little, not when we did not have much money, not when our work and travel schedules were impossible, and especially not when we were in the valleys of our married life. We kept on dating, at least every two weeks when the kids were young, and weekly now.

What do I mean by "dating," and how is it a love ritual? For starters, here is what marital dating is not: it is not going to a movie, sitting in the darkened theater, and then driving home. That's seeing a movie together, not going out on a date; you might as well have watched it at home. It is not going to dinner with another couple; that's socializing with friends, not dating each other. It is not jogging together when you enjoy each other's company but are too winded to talk; that's a recreational ritual, not a date. Do you get the picture? Dating is going out together, just the two of you, to connect emotionally through conversation and pleasurable activities.

Why does dating generally mean leaving the home? Because certain kinds of more intimate conversations happen more easily away from home. I remember Leah and me trying to have a special dinner, like on a date, when our son was a baby. We figured we would wait until he was asleep for the night before cooking our steaks, opening the bottle of Gallo Hearty Burgundy, and lighting the candles for a romantic dinner. At the first sound of clinking wine glasses as we celebrated our brilliant strategy of date-night-at-home, Eric woke up crying. We cut each other's steak as we took turns holding a squirming baby. So much for date night chez Doherty.

Here is one couple's successful date ritual still going strong nearly fifteen years into their marriage. They use payday every other week as a time to go out on a date, even if in the early years of the marriage they had only enough money for a dollar movie (the old days!) or taking a peanut-butter sandwich to the park.

They continued to do this ritual even after their special-needs child was born, viewing it as even more important than before. They don't talk about parenting or other family problems; they just focus on each other as adults and friends.

Notice the elements of this date ritual. They always went out, even if just to a park bench. They also did something pleasurable, even if was just to eat a peanut-butter sandwich or see a cheap movie. And they always talked personally, about "us," and not about logistics or family problems. They had a moment of freedom from talking about their parenting responsibilities. During these dates, they took back their marriage, for a time, from the burdens of daily life.

Sex as a Love Ritual

Sex can be lots of things other than a love ritual. It can be a physical release, an obligation, a way to make babies, a recreational activity, or even a way to control someone. To be a love ritual, sex has to have the three elements of a ritual: it has to be repeated, coordinated, and significant.

Let's start with repeated. We know that there is a steady decline in the frequency of sexual intercourse over time among all kinds of couples, likely due to familiarity and the aging process. (This occurs whether or not there are children, but the frequency of sexual relations takes a particular hit after the first child is born.) However, there is still plenty of opportunity to make sex a regular ritual in almost any couple's life. In past generations, when the cultural taboos taught that sex, even inside marriage, was a dirty activity, many spouses avoided making sex a regular love ritual for that reason. Nowadays, the consumer culture sees sex as a personal commodity to be enjoyed. We are entitled to sexual fulfillment, whether by natural means or by pharmaceutical enhancement. The danger now is that each spouse will have sex only when he or she spontaneously wants to, not when the marriage needs it.

What do I mean by the marriage needing sex? For sex to be a love bond in marriage, we have to make it a regular ritual in our relationship. Like all rituals, we hope and expect it to give us joy. But just as we should engage in affectionate greeting rituals whether or not we feel inspired at the moment, we should also approach sexual relations in the same way. It's easy for most couples to have regular sexual relations when they are young and energetic. It's harder when energies sag and life responsibilities mount. That's when it takes commitment to the relationship to keep sex a regular ritual. In consumer marriage, all it takes is for one spouse to not "feel like it" very often for the couple's sexual life to go on the shelf. Similarly, all it takes is for one spouse to find Internet pornography more attractive for the same outcome to occur. An emphasis on sexual satisfaction as personal entitlement undermines sex as a love ritual in marriage. Sometimes you do it because your marriage needs it.

If sex is to be a love ritual it must be not just repeated or regular, but also coordinated. Fortunately, there are lots of good books and videos for couples who want ideas about sex and its wonderful varieties. Here I want to focus on something simple that is not talked about very often: going to bed together. In our language, "sleeping together," or "going to bed together" are metaphors for sex. So why do so many couples not end their day in the same bed at the same time? The first phase in a dance is being on the dance floor together at the same time, next to each other. For most couples that means the bedroom at night. (Granted, if you have no children in the house, you have more options, but going to bed together at night still has special meaning for most of us.)

The culprit, once again, is the individualistic, consumerist approach to married life. If my biorhythms make me a night person and yours make you want to sleep at 10:00 P.M., I expect that each of us will do what comes naturally. Sleep is a personal thing, right? If you criticize me for hardly ever coming to bed with you, I can claim that I won't be able to go to sleep if I do. Bear in mind that I am talking here about couples who rarely end up in bed together at night, not couples where one or the other sometimes stays up after the other goes to bed.

When I counsel couples who are distant and sexless in their marriages, I ask them about their bedtime routines. For the most part, they do not go to bed together. Some of this no doubt becomes avoidance of each other, and other times sexual problems have led to safety by avoidance. But often the drift apart started innocently with a unilateral decision of one spouse, years ago, to start staying up later or going to bed earlier. Maybe it was a way to grant each other some space and privacy after busy days with work and the kids. But the pattern becomes a wedge between them in their sexual relationship, something hard to get out of because it seems unavoidable due to differences in sleep needs.

These couples are surprised when I mention the idea of going to bed together for connection, and then the night owl getting up after the other spouse has fallen asleep. You would have thought I had invented the lightbulb! It never occurs to people that the first purpose of going to bed together is to be together in physical closeness, and that sleeping is what happens next. For couples who are interested, I help them negotiate a nightly ritual of physical and verbal connection at bedtime, with sex being more of a possibility because they are coordinated enough to make it possible. If they resist getting back in touch this way, then we start addressing the deeper reasons for their lack of bedtime coordination.

Once sexual rituals become possible for couples, they can intentionally shape their sexual relationship. I remember a couple telling me about their Saturday morning ritual. Whoever woke up first (they were early risers, generally before the children woke up) would make a slow, gentle move on the one sleeping, who sometimes would pretend to still be dreaming and fantasizing about sex. Another couple signaled each other that sex tonight was going to be special by one of them lighting a special candle on the bed stand. Some couples decide to make love with their eyes open, in order to enhance their emotional and erotic connections. (Psychologist and author David Schnarch strongly recommends this practice.) Others plan couple vacations with the full intention of making lots of time to renew their sexual acquaintance with each other.

There are no rules or prescriptions for sex as a love ritual, but being mindful about this part of a marriage is terribly important. In fact, good sexual rituals keep some marriages alive during periods when the distractions of the rest of life move them in different directions.

The Difference between Love and Intimacy

Love rituals are ways to say, "I treasure you, you are my special one." But some love rituals go a step further into what I call intimacy, which occurs when the two people are open to each other in a way that is deeper and more vulnerable than we generally experience in everyday life. Intimacy rituals are love rituals where there is an element of mutual self-disclosure, where the partners come to know each other more deeply as friends and confidants. The distinction between love and intimacy can be difficult to follow. Here's an example from outside of marriage: You may love your father deeply, and show him this love in special ways, but never feel free to ask him how it feels to be getting old and having his body fail him. That kind of disclosure would be intimate, and your relationship itself would be intimate if you also felt free to tell him how it feels to have a father who is failing and will leave you before too many years. This kind of parent–child relationship is rare. Love can be strong without much in the way of intimacy.

But in marriage, most couples born in the psychological era of the second half of the twentieth century want not just love, but also give-and-take emotional intimacy. It's just that this kind of intimacy is hard to find in marriage, and occurs rarely unless we create ritual possibilities for it to occur. Intimacy rituals are a staple of courtship for many couples, but a golden achievement after years of marriage.

An example of an intimate conversation is the mutual sharing of hopes and dreams for the future. A woman once told me that she used to love the long walks she and her fiancé would take, during which he would talk about the future he aspired to for himself and their future family, and she would do the same. She especially treasured the conversations in which he reflected on how the death of his father at a young age had made it hard for him to find his path as a man in the world. Now that he had found his love mate, he said he felt empowered to forge that path. But married for nine years now, with two children, they had long ago ceased having those kinds of conversations.

Understanding why intimacy is difficult in marriage is one of the most important things any of us can learn. Unless we understand it, we are not inclined to create love rituals and intimacy rituals. Unless we understand it, we are vulnerable to be attracted to new romantic partners with whom we can re-create a golden age of emotional intimacy, only to lose it again if we marry that person. Intimacy is challenging in marriage because, in the furnace of a marriage relationship, it takes a high degree of self-definition (self-differentiation, to use the technical term) to stay connected while holding on to yourself. You have to know who you are, know what you feel, and say what you want to maintain your psychological boundaries in marriage. This is especially difficult in times of conflict and when we feel anxious and rejected by our mate. Think of the range of reactions people have when their husband or wife does not want to have sex with them.

Let's go back to the metaphor of you and your mate in a canoe. When you were on the shore, talking openly about your past boating experiences and your dreams for being on the river together, it was relatively easy to be open and to listen to the other's honest words. Once you are in the boat together and hit the first rapids, it becomes harder to be open to your mate's comments about your poor paddling technique and about whether you should have entered the river at a different location, and about why you forgot to pack the insect repellent. On top of that, your spouse is getting tired of all the rowing, and his or her shoulder is aching; can you do more on your own, please? In other words, when you enter the interdependent world of marriage, the stakes are higher, the anxiety is greater, the conflicts more intense, the heat of love and hate greater. It takes a lot of psychological maturity to keep your balance. When we fear losing our balance—ourselves, really—and when we have trouble trusting that our spouse will accept our innermost feelings, worries, and hopes, then we clog up the well of intimate self-disclosure. We may still love deeply, and say so regularly, but we are afraid to share what is most personal.

I am not going to say anything magical to help you grow personally in your ability to be intimate with your mate. It's a lifelong journey for all of us. What I do want to talk about is creating rituals where intimate encounters become safer and more likely to occur.

Intimacy Rituals

After this buildup about intimacy, I hope you do not think that intimacy rituals have to be as grand as the Mars space probe. In fact, intimacy cannot be manufactured by a ritual or any other means. All you can do is set the scene and hope that the atmosphere is conducive. It's like humor; you can't force it. Here is a small example from my dates with Leah. We especially like to go out to dinner together, sometimes after a movie. We have always had two favorite restaurants at a time, one for special occasions and one for regular dining out. (We go to other restaurants, too, but tend to gravitate back to our favorites.)

Sometimes, I will decide to ask Leah one of the big questions that people who are becoming close like to ask each other, along the lines of: How do you see your life now that the kids are gone and self-supporting? Or, what do you see yourself doing in five years? Or, did you ever think you would have so much success when you started making jewelry? Or, what are you looking forward to next year? Or, how do you feel about both of us getting older?

Reading these questions on paper can make them sound like interview questions, but I think they instead express my interest in knowing what is going on inside Leah, how she is feeling about herself and her life. These are the sorts of questions that couples don't often take the time to ask each other. And then, if she signals an interest in talking, I sit back and listen. She has my full attention, and I am often surprised by something she says that I did not know before. This kind of listening requires relaxation on the listener's part, a readiness to ask follow-up questions, to empathize with what the other person is saying, and most of all, to settle in to hear the full story. (If you analyze the responses, or disagree with them, your spouse will likely shut down.) Sometimes Leah follows up with similar questions to me. Sometimes we will both share our thoughts on what it feels like to be at a similar stage of life, when our parents are gone and our children have mates and children of their own—and when we lose friends to illness on a disturbingly frequent basis. Or about our own future together.

One of the paradoxes of married life, after the first couple of honeymoon years, is that we generally stop asking each other and telling each other about important personal matters such as these. It's as if we stand too close together to really see each other as fully separate people. We assume we understand and then lose our curiosity about the mystery of our partner. Perhaps the problem is that we are afraid of what the answers might be, or that our spouse might see us as intrusive. Whatever the reason, most of us don't inquire about the kinds of things we would ask a friend whom we see from time to time, such as "How is your work really going for you?" and "What does it feel like to turn fifty?" and "How are you handling not being able to run any more because of your knee problem?" If you want to ask these kinds of intimate questions, you can try to lead up to them rather than spring them. For example, you can wait for a quiet, alone time when your spouse is talking about the joys or stresses of work to ask the work question. You can ask the "fifty-year-old" question during a private birthday dinner after you have wished your mate a happy birthday. And the key is not the opening question but your loving interest in going wherever your spouse wants to take the conversation.

As I said, these rituals of intimacy are fragile and cannot be forced. A bad waiter or a too-noisy restaurant can douse the mood. Sometimes a short but thoughtfully considered "I don't know" response can lead to more reflection and a later intimate conversation.

Love rituals and intimacy rituals are like regular sex and special sex; the first is a familiar and reliable companion, the second you can get yourself prepared for but always feels like a gift.

When I wrote these words for the first edition of this book, I felt more vulnerable than about anything else in the book—not vulnerable so much to the readers, but to Leah, who would soon look at these words as my first reader. I had never made explicit to her before what I sometimes intentionally do to connect more deeply with her. Intimacy rituals are delicate things. As I came to find out, she knew all along what I was doing.

Love Rituals of Remembrance and Security

Later, when we talk about anniversaries and other special occasions, I will give more examples of other spoken intimacy rituals. But for now, I would like to end our discussion of love rituals with two of my favorites from couples who have attended my workshops. I'll paraphrase and change a bit of the content to protect their privacy. Margaret was barely sixteen years old when she and Terry, age eighteen, began dating. He was a high school dropout with little to show for himself except a fancy imported convertible. They would sometimes ride all night in his convertible with the top down, and they still like to ride together in the dark thirty-five years later. They had sex together for the first time in that convertible, and Margaret reports that they have made love in every car they've owned since!

The final love ritual reminds me that rituals can be healing as well as being expressions of connection and love. Louise and Mark's ritual began shortly after Louise was raped. It was early in their married life. As a nurse, Louise works odd shifts, including evenings and some early mornings when it's still dark. She began to call her husband when she arrived at work and when she was about to leave for home. At first, this was mainly for a sense of security, for both of them, but eventually they both came to realize that it allowed them both the chance to say, "I love you," and for Louise to begin to refocus her day from work to home. They never, ever fail to have that phone call and to end it with those words.

I don't know about you, but I have tears in my eyes now. I feel touched and inspired by the stories that couples have shared with me, and I feel close to the sacred core of the marriage crucible, which, if we let it, has the power to heal us and transform us.

Moving from inspiration to actually putting more love rituals into your relationship, of course, requires careful planning and timing. In the last chapter in the book, I will tell you about some different ways to start. In the meantime, let's move on to anniversary rituals and other special occasions for couples.

10 Intentional Marriage
Anniversaries and Other Special Occasions

Married life is a daily thing, which is its joy and its downfall. Special occasion rituals like anniversaries and birthdays and Valentine's Day allow us to punctuate the run-on sentence of daily life. We stop to hold up our loved one and our marriage to a bright light, apart from the logistics and schedules of the rest of life. We say special things that would become trite if we said them every day. We give special gifts that would overwhelm our budgets or our imaginations if we gave them every month. In these bracketed moments of special intensity, we acknowledge what is unique and irreplaceable about our marriage. We mark the passage of another year in each other's lives. It was during an anniversary ritual one year that I realized that I had been married to Leah for more than half of my life, and noted that to her. She realized the same was true for her. We shook our heads with disbelief and looked into each other's eyes. When else do you get to say that kind of thing and have that kind of shared experience? Let's talk about the rituals of anniversaries and special occasions.

Wedding Anniversaries

Wedding anniversaries are a ritual opportunity with great untapped potential for many couples. When I ask people about their anniversary celebrations, they generally respond with an embarrassed laugh, saying that they spend it doing things like watching their child's soccer game or cleaning up the backyard. Yes, there is a lot of untapped potential for most of us.

Almost everyone makes a big deal of their first few anniversaries, but after that, many couples put energy only into the big ones of twenty-five and fifty, if they live that long. Family and friends don't track your wedding anniversary like they do your birthday, so there is not a lot of discussion about its coming up on the schedule. Your kids, until they are older and start thinking about marriage themselves, couldn't care less about your anniversary. What's more, anniversaries are inconvenient because they fall on any old day of the work week.

But more than anything else, many of us don't make a fuss over our anniversaries because we have long ago stopped making a fuss over our relationships. Our attention is elsewhere. We still love each other and may be good partners in life's tasks, but we have grown accustomed to the slow drift south. But even if one of us gets inspired to pull out more stops for our next anniversary, we may not have a lot of imagination left about what to do. If we do not have regular connection and love rituals, including dates, then we may not know how to have a meaningful anniversary ritual; it's like we are out of practice. And some years one or both of us may forget that our anniversary is upon us, whereupon we let it go or scramble to do something, anything.

If you feel good about your anniversary ritual, then tell others about it so that they can be inspired. If you need inspiration yourself, then learn about couples like Steve and Luanne, who rescued their anniversary from ritual oblivion. Their anniversary was Christmas. So they always lost their anniversary to the holidays. And then they had a child born on Christmas. So Steve decided to save their anniversary by "kidnapping" Luanne and take her somewhere. All he says is take your clothes and your coat, and come with me. He has a limo outside and they go off somewhere fun. They take back their anniversary!

Notice how the deck was originally stacked against this couple's anniversary by its time in the year. I'll bet that their family and friends also lost track of their anniversary in the Christmas and birthday rush every year. Then Steve stepped up to the plate one year, for reasons I do not know, and hit a home run for the anniversary, probably without intending to repeat the performance every year. But the anniversary "kidnapping" became an annual ritual of renewal and recommitment by which they define what is special about their marriage. In fact, Steve and Luanne did something that researchers in recent years have paid attention to: the power of surprise events to build intimacy in couples. It's a nice complement to regular, predictable rituals: spicing up the relationship with something novel.

Okay, so you don't have the wherewithal to rent a limo, leave town, and have someone watch your children. That's not really the point. All it takes to have an intentional anniversary ritual is to believe it is important, plan ahead, and do something special as a couple. Whatever is special to the two of you. But it does require leadership for your marriage, not staying on automatic pilot.

Dick and Kathy don't do anything spectacular with their anniversary, except for acknowledging it every month! They were married on August 22, and they celebrate their monthly wedding anniversary on the twenty-second. They do something special, although not necessarily something big or expensive. It might be going out to dinner, or just a phone call and "Happy Anniversary, I love you," or leaving a note in the morning. They have kept this anniversary ritual alive, at last count, for four hundred thirty months!

If you do the math, you will see that Dick and Kathy have been married for nearly thirty-six years. Their anniversary ritual is a beacon for their life together. In their words, "We try to keep it alive." That could be the motto for the intentional, committed-for-the-long-haul marriage.

At this moment, my mind goes to my parents' marriage. Like most kids, I didn't pay any attention to their anniversary; their solid marriage was a "given" in my life, something to be counted on but not commented on. I never knew that they marked the day until after my father died in 1984. Months later, when visiting my mother, I noticed that she had framed and displayed two recent anniversary cards from my father. The cards had a prominent place in the main bedroom that my mother had vacated so that Leah and I could sleep there. I don't know what else my parents did for their anniversary, but seeing these lovely cards, the last two of their married life, reminded me that we never know which anniversary will be our last one.

It's hard to keep writing after that story, but I want to tell you about how Leah and I have celebrated our anniversary. For most of our marriage, it was not a pretty picture. We got married on August 14, 1971. Mid-August is not a great time for an anniversary, I can tell you. It seemed like we spent most anniversaries in a moving van, as we relocated around the country to graduate school and various university jobs. We always moved in August, mid-August to be exact. If we were not moving, it seems that we were in a car with children, traipsing around the country visiting relatives or being on vacation. As Leah sometimes puts it, we celebrated most of our first fifteen anniversaries in a Motel 6 with a U-Haul truck outside and two squirrelly children in the next bed. Or, I would add, at a relative's house packed to the gills with family and with two squirrelly children in the next bed.

Once we settled in Minnesota in 1986 (moving in mid-August, of course), we stopped moving and we stopped taking vacations and visiting family at that time of year. Now we had to figure out how to celebrate our anniversary! We settled into a ritual of going out to whatever was our favorite special-occasions restaurant at the time. An important adjustment we made was to do this anniversary ritual at a time that was best for us, and not necessarily on the day itself. Sometimes it's stressful for couples with children to dash home from work, hope that the babysitter can still come on a weeknight, and charge off to have a romantic dinner. You can acknowledge the day itself in other ways, and then wait until the weekend to dress up and celebrate.

I learned about this kind of flexibility with family rituals from Leah's family, who would sometimes "do Christmas" anytime between Thanksgiving and Christmas when the clan could gather in one place from different parts of the country. Tree, gifts, turkey—the whole nine yards—on December 10 or 14. The idea is to get everyone there in celebration; the date is less important.

About fifteen years ago, I suggested to Leah that we add something to our anniversary dinner ritual. We had been wishing each other a happy anniversary during our dinner celebration, usually with a toast, but I felt the need for something more personal. A week or so before our anniversary one year, I proposed that, at our anniversary dinner, we each share some words of appreciation for being married to each other, something to honor and acknowledge our marriage. Leah readily agreed. A day beforehand, I reminded her about the new part of the ritual and suggested that we do it right after we got our wine.

The addition of this small ritual has deepened our anniversary by adding words of emotional intimacy. Sometimes we offer an appreciation from the previous year of our marriage, and sometimes we express wonder and gratitude for being married to each other for these now-long years. Sometimes we also share words of gratitude for changes we are still making and growth we are still experiencing. (I'll leave out the specifics because rituals like this lose something when they are too public.)

You may ask why it is necessary to have a planned ritual of intimate words between two people married this long. Why not express these sentiments spontaneously? It isn't necessary to create a ritual like this, but it sure is helpful. Otherwise, when is the right moment to open your heart in gratitude for your mate and your marriage? On a Saturday morning sometime, while your spouse is reading the paper? After lovemaking, when your heart is full and your words poetic but your spouse is already falling gently asleep?

Timing is an important reason why rituals can set us free to be intimate. If only one of you is prepared to share your deepest feelings at a particular moment, the other is likely to not know what to say in response. Your mate has rehearsed tender words of love, perhaps putting them into iambic pentameter, and then springs them on you during the appetizer course of your anniversary dinner, or on some other occasion of your mate's choosing. You feel touched, and then you realize that you've got to say something back. You mumble something like, "Me too. I love you too." Hours later, you think of what you could have said from your heart. It's not that this was a bad moment in your marriage—far from it—but it lacked the depth and mutuality that a coordinated ritual could have given you.

Instead, I suggest that you talk in advance about whether you want to have a ritual exchange of appreciation as part of your anniversary or some other ritual. If you both agree, then remind each other before the actual event, and decide when exactly you want to do it, so that neither of you is caught by surprise when the other launches. Lack of coordination here can undermine the ritual, as when your spouse says, "Can we wait a minute? I don't want this soup to get cold." That's the equivalent, for verbal expressions of intimacy, of being asked to hold off lovemaking until halftime of the football game. As I mentioned earlier in the chapter, I suggested that we do our exchange of appreciation early in the meal, when we first have a glass of wine in our hands. I am usually feeling too much emotional anticipation to wait until I am eating my entrée. So at the start, we toast each other and our marriage, and then say what is in our hearts this year about us. We each listen deeply to the other, one at a time, with no discussion of the fine points—just a ritual sharing. And then, with light hearts, we relish our anniversary meal.

For big anniversaries, or even for regular ones, consider taking a trip away together. Nothing rejuvenates marriages more than extended time away together. In fact, this is a good test of whether there is still fire in the belly of your marriage: Do you enjoy each other more, and argue less, when you take time away together? Do you make love more, and enjoy it more? Do you laugh more? (If you don't, it doesn't mean your marriage is doomed, but it probably does mean you have to work harder at it, and maybe get help to deal with conflicts that are getting in your way.) Even proposing an anniversary trip is a romantic thing to do, and a sign of leadership for your marriage. Notice that I called it an anniversary getaway, rather than a vacation that happens to fall on your anniversary. Remember Beverly and Tom's story? Their annual anniversary kidnap/getaway may also be a vacation, but as an anniversary celebration it no doubt gives them enough fuel to last the rest of the winter and through the spring. For our fortieth anniversary, Leah and I decided to make a year's worth of trips: our greatest hits, if you will—the places in the U.S. and around the world that have been special to us. This anniversary seemed too big for just one celebration. I know that my own parents' fortieth was their last big wedding anniversary before my father's death several years later. You never know.

I also talked before about making your anniversary rituals more public. There are many stakeholders in our marriages, people who benefit from our unions and help us in return. Why not get a larger community involved in the birthdays of our marriages? The reason my parents' fortieth is memorable to me is that we celebrated it as an extended family. I will return to this idea later when I talk about community support for marriage.

Valentine's Day

When I knew I had to write about Valentine's Day for the first edition of this book, I was worried. So I asked Leah for advice. She suggested that I tell the truth: that I didn't think much of Valentine's Day as a ritual occasion. It has become a commercialized cultural ritual for new lovers who enjoy the thrill of discovering that they are each other's true Valentines. As exciting as new love is, it doesn't hold a candle to marital love. And Valentine's Day is a culturally imposed time to express romantic love, which can certainly create complications.

My resistance to Valentine's Day was probably like that of many people to rituals in general. The downside of rituals is that, if we are committed to them, they can feel compulsory, something imposed on us, instead of freely chosen. We may then resent having to do the ritual and want to free ourselves from its bonds. Lots of spouses I've worked with, especially men, resist all types of marital rituals because, they say, it's better to be spontaneous. Underneath, they are saying that they don't want to be controlled by a schedule of times to connect with their mate, and underneath that, they are saying that they don't want to feel controlled by their wives. When I think about my resistance to Valentine's Day, I can sympathize with those who don't like to feel compelled by rituals, but being a conscientious objector to all marital rituals leads, in most cases, not to more spontaneous connection, but to little connection at all.

I do want to underline, however, that after boycotting Valentine's Day for many years and not giving Leah any acknowledgment—card, flowers, or candy—I came to believe that it is important to recognize the day. When the whole culture is talking about romantic love for a day, ideological objections no longer keep me from acknowledging my own sweetie. I now plan a month or two in advance by booking a reservation at a romantic restaurant that fills up quickly on Valentine's Day. And we have a lovely, if usually low-key, time. I've come to enjoy the presence of mainly couples (not big dinner parties) around us, and their quiet conversations.

If you really don't like the compulsory nature of Valentine's Day rituals, you don't have to do them, although you risk hurting your mate's feelings. But you might want to consider going with the cultural flow and making the day your own, like the choice to get into the spirit of Christmas (for those who celebrate this holiday) by deciding it's better to use it as a time to connect instead of abstaining and waiting for a more spontaneous day or season.

Birthdays

Birthday rituals can be a reminder that every marriage is a cross-cultural experience, even if you marry the kid next door. The reason? We marry outside of our families, and every family has its own culture. Birthdays were a big deal in my family, but only until you became an adult, at which time birthdays were acknowledged only with a card. We didn't celebrate my parents' birthdays at all. Again, for me, birthday rituals were very important for kids, but not for adults.

But in Leah's family, birthday celebrations were a big ritual for all ages. Everyone knew everyone else's birthdays—children, parents, grandparents, aunts, uncles, cousins, and neighbors. And they all—I mean everyone—showed up for everyone else's birthday parties. Let the good times roll. Leah entered marriage with high expectations for birthdays.

You can see where this is heading. Leah went all out for my birthdays, which I thought was nice but perhaps a bit excessive. But it took me many years before I got my mind around the fact that I should do something really special for Leah's birthdays. I know, you are wondering why I was so dense. Every year I would not think about her approaching birthday until it was upon us, and after she reminded me, and then I would come through with a present and celebration that were, shall I say, less than thrilling. Leah was gracious about what I did for her birthday, but not amused by my forgetfulness and last-minute efforts. Sometimes she told me that she felt hurt. After being defensive for a while, I would come to recognize that I had let her down, acknowledge this to her, and resolve to do better next year. But a year is a long time to remember a resolution, at least for me, especially when I did not yet emotionally understand what she was talking about. Birthdays were for kids.

I don't remember when I began to get it, but I know it was only in the 1990s. I am not a quick study in these matters, I guess. But I came to see Leah's birthday as a way to extend myself for her. I learned that it is pleasurable for both of us if I plan months in advance for what I will do for her birthday. I try to get her one present that will knock her socks off. It took me more than twenty years, but I learned to use my wife's birthday as a time to do something truly special for her. I see it as my time to give back, in a visible and tangible way, for what she gives me so bountifully the rest of the year. I want her to feel touched, to feel special and cherished. That's a goal that I now enjoy trying to reach. I still don't see my own birthday as such a big deal, but I have learned to embrace this difference.

I want to stress that going over the top on birthday rituals does not have to mean spending a lot of money. It's how well the ritual is suited to your mate, and how much love and sensitivity it carries. One husband I know always takes off work on his wife's birthday and plans a day of fun activities. He calls her friends and coworkers to remind them of her birthday. He does these things because he knows that for his wife, her birthday is the high point of the year.

Be Creative with Your Own Special Rituals

Married couples, I have found, are enormously creative in developing special-occasion rituals that would never occur to me. One couple I know makes a big, personal deal over New Year's Eve, whereas others just try to stay off the streets. Although Christmas is mainly a family ritual, some couples find a special moment on Christmas Eve to celebrate their love. Even rituals for children, such as a birthday or a Bar Mitzvah, can be occasions for carving out a special time for couple connection by noting and celebrating the miracle that your marriage brought this growing child into the world. I even know an American couple who celebrate Bastille Day every year.

When couples tell me about how they make rituals of their special occasions, and when I think of Leah's and mine, I sense an undercurrent of healthy marital pride. Marital pride? We talk about proud parents but not about proud couples, except maybe pride in being married for many years. Creating special rituals just for you and your mate, being committed to these rituals year after year, and nurturing them to keep them fresh—these are ways to punctuate the daily routines of your life together with occasional exclamation points and to grow a sense of fulsome pride in your marriage.

11 Every Marriage Supported by a Community

To paraphrase the poet John Donne, no marriage is an island, apart from the shore. Who among us has not felt the painful loss of friends' marriages, where we first lose our ties with them as a couple and then with one or both of them as individuals? The longer we have known this marriage, the more unsettling the divorce. Marriages are like trees in the town square. The big, long-lived oaks, when they become uprooted, take large hunks of community property with them.

At first, we commiserate with both divorcing parties, and we say that we don't want to take sides. But it rarely works out that way. One of the spouses calls us more frequently, asking for emotional support. We hear one side of the divorce more than the other. The other person knows this, and drifts away. Even the friend we keep may move gradually into a different social world.

Divorcing spouses carve up their community like they do their property. She gets the church, and he keeps the bowling league. She keeps the couple of friends from her work setting, and he keeps the ones from his work. After twenty years of asking your friend Mary how her husband, Fred, is, you must never ask again. He is dead to you. To quote novelist Judith Guest, "Every divorce is the death of a small civilization." Marriage is not just a private relationship in an individualistic, consumer society; it is also a public bond between two citizens of a community.

If we agree to be stakeholders in one another's marriages, sometimes the support we offer or receive is not going to be of the "feel-good" variety. Sometimes it will come in the form of stubborn refusal to give up on someone's marriage. One group of twelve couples who socialized together for many years and grew to know one another's marriages without a lot of explicit talk about their relationships, faced the prospect of the divorce of one of the couples. The other couples rallied, talked extensively with both spouses, got them to a good therapist, and nurtured them through their crisis to a better relationship beyond. Weren't they being intrusive? You bet. The phrase they used was, "We don't want to lose one of our own." Just as they had done for couples who faced physical illness, this group rallied around a couple facing a marital illness. Instead of stepping back and just saying, "It's a private matter" or "It's their choice," they held the couple up until they healed. They helped their friends and community members cling as a couple until the new glue could congeal.

Sadly, most of us are not fortunate enough to have this kind of community. I remember the moment when I realized this about my own marriage. I was driving down a freeway toward a meeting. I asked myself two questions. The first was "Who are the people who have helped me be a parent, people who have helped me raise my children?" The car was suddenly filled with the faces of people—relatives, teachers, friends—who had directly helped me and Leah to raise Eric and Elizabeth into adulthood, people who knew us well as parents and knew our children well. I remember, for example, the crucial support we received from parents at our church while we were adjusting to having babies in our lives. It came mostly in the form of caring gestures and of words like, "We've been there, it's hard right now, but your baby is magnificent!" We had many stakeholders in our parenting.

Then I asked a second question: "Who has helped me to grow my marriage, people who have known my marriage well?" The car suddenly emptied of faces, to be replaced by a few shadowy ones. Yes, I knew that many people had cared about the success of our marriage. But who, I wondered, had directly supported us and known us as married people the way that they had supported and known us as parents? It was a hard question to answer, and left me feeling uneasy.

I thought that maybe it was my lack of imagination or memory, so that night I asked Leah the same question. She also drew a blank, thinking of people who have indirectly supported our marriage because they have supported us as individuals or as parents, but not people who have understood our marriage well and helped us directly. For example, I can never remember anyone asking how Leah and I were handling some part of our marital life together. Nor, outside of my professional role as a therapist, have I very often asked a similar question of a friend—unless there was an obvious source of stress such as a serious illness in one of the spouses.

I invite you to do the same self-examination I have done about the community base of my own marriage. You may find it a hard question to understand. At one level, if you have a good number of people who support you in your life, then of course they support your marriage. And studies show that couples with an overlapping circle of friends—in other words, good friends in common—have more satisfied marriages. But mostly this is indirect support. Ask yourself about whether anyone has mentored you as a married person the way someone might have in your job. Ask yourself about how often you trade stories of strategies, successes, and failures about other aspects of life—parenting, jobs, personal health—versus how often you trade similar stories about your marriage. If you feel well supported in your community, I am glad for you. If you don't, you are part of a very large club.

The problem here is a cultural assumption that we live our married lives largely by ourselves. Instead of community-based marriage, we have solitary marriage. The pioneer marriage educator and counselor David Mace called it the "intermarital taboo," the fear of asking about or revealing what goes on inside our marital relationships. A woman who will ask her friend the most intimate details about becoming a mother—Did they do an episiotomy? Did your milk come without difficulty?—would probably be reluctant to ask a tame question such as whether she and her husband are getting any time to be a couple now that they are parents. Partly this reticence is because a marriage is a two-way relationship; asking about a marriage is asking about the mate, not just the friend.

But most of us feel free to ask about dating relationships, or an ill spouse. But marriage is a zone of privacy—and isolation.

We begin our marriages with loads of social support. That's what wedding rituals are for. Weddings are the historical way in which the stakeholders in a marriage come together in support of it.

Many religious congregations are now requiring premarital preparation, which is an additional form of support for the new marriage. The only other marital event that is universally acknowledged by a community is the death of one of the spouses. A wedding to launch a marriage, a funeral to end it—the rest of the time you are on your own as far as your community is concerned.

It is not uncommon for individual spouses, particularly wives, to talk to friends about their marriages. This can be an important form of support, if your friends care about your marriage as well as you personally. (We talked about that before.) A number of research studies have shown that when women who are happy with their marriages confide in friends about problems in the marriage, they often come away with a more balanced perspective and stronger positive feelings toward their husbands. (Men confide less often about their marriages.) But when you talk individually with friends, they get only your perspective on your marriage and its challenges. Chances are, you and your mate as a couple are open about your marriage with exactly no one. If you are open in this way, I would like you to write to me so that I can learn more about how you managed to overcome the cultural norm that inner life of a marriage is a game of solitaire for two.

Why Solitary Marriage Is a Problem

Most of the couples I see as a marital therapist don't realize how common their problems are. They get demoralized because they think they are alone in their lapses and frustrations. It would be like young parents bringing their two-year-old to a child psychologist because the child has started to scream "NO" and throw tantrums. Without frank discussion in family and friendship circles about the normal phases and strains of married life, many couples think their marriage is in the bottom two percent instead of squarely at the fiftieth percentile. Or they don't realize that in one area they are far below the norm, but that in another they lead the pack. Take the pursuer–distancer pattern that we discussed before. It is nearly universal in married life. Or differences in handling feelings about the serious illness of a loved one. Or feeling more disconnected as a couple during the intense time of raising infants and toddlers. One problem with solitary marriage is that people don't know what comes with the territory of being married today, versus what is beyond the pale.

A second problem with solitary marriage is that people don't have access to the wisdom of other couples who have faced obstacles and either overcome them or learned to live with them gracefully. It's one thing to read books by experts about marriage, and it's another thing to hear it from a peer or elder who has walked in your shoes. Even if you have to adapt the wisdom and advice to your own situation because your marriage or age is different, you are apt to learn something and be inspired. Do you remember learning and feeling inspired by the rituals that couples shared with us earlier in this book? They shared their insights at a conference for couples. I want to tell you the opening story at my presentation at that conference, as an illustration of what we can learn if we are open with one another about our marriages:

> "I had a fascinating conversation with the taxi driver on the way from the airport to this conference. When he mentioned his wife, I asked him how long he had been married. 'Forty-seven years married,' he said, 'and I'm sixty-eight years old.' He was an African American gentleman who seemed to be in great physical shape. I asked him about his secret of his marital longevity. Without hesitation, he replied: 'Get things out in the open. No secrets. When you have a fight, you have to make up afterwards. Which means someone has to apologize first.' He added that he always apologizes first. This guy's been reading the marriage research, or maybe he doesn't have to. He then ventured into the domain of gender roles. He recounted the time

when one of his ten grandchildren asked him, 'Grandpa, are you the head of the family?' He answered slowly and carefully, 'Yes, I guess I am, but if I'm the head, Grandma's the neck, and you know, the head never moves without the neck moving first.'"

I felt like I had already attended the most interesting talk of the conference, before I even got to the hotel. Every couple has something to teach if we find the vehicle.

A third problem with solitary marriage is that couples suffer alone when they are in distress. How often have you been surprised and pained to learn that a friend or loved one has announced a divorce, when you never knew they were having problems? With the same couples, if one of them had cancer you would have known about it. If one of them had a dying parent or sick child, you would have known about it. The couple's community, of which you are a part, probably would have rallied in the support. But so often couples suffer in public silence as their demoralization grows, ashamed to say anything now and unaccustomed to saying anything at all. How do you all of a sudden open up about your growing marital crisis when you have not talked about the smaller problems? Again, one of the spouses might talk to a friend before the breakup, but research studies have found that distressed spouses talk more often to single, divorced, and unhappily married friends and don't get a lot of supportive and validating comments about the marriage. Meanwhile, the couple often keeps up appearances for their couple friends.

A fourth problem is that, even when couples seek counseling, there is too much pressure on the counseling alone if the couple do not have adequate support in their community. Sam Gurnoe, an American Indian healer and family therapist, once said something to a group of therapists that I have never forgotten. In making a distinction between the benefits of therapy and the deep healing that only comes within a community, he said, "Outside of a community, a culture, and a spirituality, you can treat but you cannot heal." He went on to say that he is not against treatment. It is important and can do good. But he was calling us to the realization that true healing is sustained in the embrace of a community larger than a specific individual, marriage, or family. In therapy, we try to create a small healing community in the office, only to send couples out to play solitaire again after we finished our work with them.

Marriage Was Not Always So Solitary

Nothing about marriage was as private in the past as almost everything is now, even sexual relations, because most families slept together in large rooms. Until the nineteenth century, family life in Europe and North America was focused outward toward the community rather than inward toward the nuclear family. Housing was dark and cramped, so families spent as much time outdoors as possible, which meant in the public view. Most people were born, married, raised children, and died within one geographical community. They knew many others and were known. They married someone they and their family had known all their lives. When serious marital problems arose, other people knew about it. In Puritan New England, we know that, in the case of severe marital problems such as physical abuse and infidelity, the village elders would pay visits to the offending spouse in order to bring him or her back into conformity with community standards.

In New Mexican Hispanic villages prior to the nineteenth century, there was a system of support for couples and families. There were *compadrazgo,* people who assisted the family in the ceremonies associated with the rites of passage. We are all familiar with the traditional role of godparents, who not only assisted with the baptism but also had responsibility for the moral upbringing of the child. Only recently did I become aware, through the writing of historian Adrian Bustamante, of "marriage godparents" in New Mexican Hispanic culture. Termed *padrinos de boda,* marriage godparents were responsible not only for helping with the prescribed wedding rituals but also for counseling their *ahijados* (godchildren) if they encountered marital difficulties.

Even today, in many non-Western cultures there is more community support for marriage than in our culture. The African American writer Sobonfu Some has written about marriage in her home village in West Africa, where marriage is not considered just a private relationship. She reports that, when a couple are in marital distress, the whole village knows it and is affected by it. The social well-being of the village is affected when a marriage goes bad. And there are prescribed ways to intervene to help the couple. The women talk to the wife, and the men talk to the husband. If that is not successful, then representatives of the women and men come together to mediate the conflict. Can you see how the positive social pressure mounts to overcome your marital problems? Your marital happiness and unhappiness are not just your own in a communal culture. Finally, when the couple reconciles, they go through a ritual of purification and reconnection in the river, where the spouses are separately put under water by members of their own gender, after which they join hands under the water and emerge together, hands held high, to the applause and rejoicing of the village.

We can't hold a candle to this kind of support for marriage. Our culture is too individualistic, too oriented to privacy and autonomy.

A year ago, I performed a wedding for two dear friends. (In their state, a layperson can perform a wedding by going through certain application procedures.) At the wedding, I asked the guests to think about how they would support the commitment and the relationship of this couple. And then, with a hand-held microphone, I moved around the room inviting the family and loved ones of the couple to express this promise out loud to the couple. It was quite powerful, ranging from promises to pray for the couple to a guarantee from one big, burly, and kindly man that he would "kick [the husband's] butt" if he did not treat his new wife as well as she deserved. As wonderful as this ritual of community was, I later realized that without clear ways to make this support happen, it may have offered little more than good intentions.

What You and Your Spouse Can Do

I want to come clean with you. I still don't have a community-based marriage myself, and I am only beginning to learn what one would look like. Of all the things I have written about in this book, this is the most underdeveloped.

Following are some things you can try personally to promote community-based marriage for yourself and others in your life. These are in addition to being part of the community-level initiatives I will outline later. None of them are easy, given the privacy taboo about marriage. But they are places to start.

• Be more open about your marriage with people who are close to you. If this is new to you, be careful to start slowly, with routine matters like how much time you have for each other these days, as opposed to starting with your on-and-off-again sex life!

• Ask people about their marriages. Again, you don't have to start "heavy." You can ask about how they met; most people love to tell that story. When a couple has been through a transition like having a first child, you can ask whether they are getting any time for themselves. (And you can offer to babysit so that they can get out.) When a couple's last child has left home, you can ask what it's like now. When you talk to a couple married for many years, ask for their secret of longevity; they will be glad to tell you.

• Pay people compliments about their marriage when you see things you like. I am struck with how rarely most of us hear positive comments about our marriages. It's a way of saying we notice and value this important area of people's lives.

• If you and your spouse are close to another couple, bring up the idea of the four of you checking in with each other about your marriages. It would bring a deeper intimacy to your friendship and serve as a sounding board for your couple relationships. A good time to do this would be if all four of you have participated in the next idea below.

• Go to marriage education and enrichment events. These are places to meet other couples who are interested in growing their marriages and in giving and receiving support. Speak up at one of these events to ask whether other couples are interested in meeting to talk about your marriages. Having shared the same marriage education experience can give you and other couples a common vocabulary to talk about marriage. To repeat, don't miss an opportunity to be involved publicly in marriage-related events in your community, because there the ice has already been broken and there you will find kindred spirits.

What Communities Can Do

Now let's talk about what communities can do to support marriage. Of course, communities can do nothing unless we as individuals take the initiative. One of the early themes in our discussion about marriage was the idea of being a citizen of one's marriage. Here I want to expand the idea to that of community citizenship for marriage. Think of the communities you are a part of, where you might be able to broach the idea of a community initiative for marriage, or where you might join one that others start.

I think that community initiatives will occur most readily in already existing communities, like religious communities, or in institutions that already have the confidence of their communities, such as the YMCA, family service agencies, Jewish community centers, and family education centers. Although it is possible that neighborhood associations and other loosely affiliated groups might spring up around marriage, I am more hopeful that centers that already have a structure and community trust are the places to start. Some of them will have to decide first that marriage is an important part of their mission. I won't try to convince them here, but I will talk about what they can do once they decide that support for marriage is a high priority. Remember, the "they" in this case is you and I as well, because we are members of these institutions and citizens of these communities.

• Create mentor couple programs of the kind that are springing up in religious communities around the country. This initiative has been led by people such as Mike and Harriet McManus and Leslie and Leslie Parrott. Mentor couples generally have ten or more years in marriages that both spouses regard, and their community regards, as successful. They receive training in how to support and guide younger couples, especially those just entering marriages.

Then they are matched with these couples, with an expectation of meeting several times a year for several years. This kind of mentoring creates stakeholders in other people's marriages, and benefits both the new couple and the mentor couple. Lest you think that newlyweds don't need support because they are in the bloom of love, remember that there are many couples whose parachute never opens, who falter right away and have nowhere to turn.

• Bring together couples for crisis help. A pastor tells the story of asking, during his sermon, for couples to meet him in a church room after the service if they have had a time of serious difficulty in their marriage and have come out the other side, and if they would like to help other couples who are now in crisis. A larger than expected number of couples showed up, including many whose crises he had been blind to. They received training to serve as helpers for couples in serious trouble, with great success, from what I am told. This help is not inconsistent with marital therapy; in fact, it could be a terrific adjunct to professional help.

• Create cluster groups of couples for support and outreach. Instead of traditional support groups, where people tend to "consume" the support of the group until they don't need it anymore, I recommend groups that have dual missions: to support one another in their marriages and to do good for other marriages in the communities. I know such a group of African American couples who have formed a covenant to support one another's marriages and reach out to the community. They have developed an innovative way to get to know one another's marriage more deeply. Each couple declares three areas of the relationship they want to work on and improve, and they give the okay for others in the group to check in with them on a regular basis about how they are progressing in that area. The beauty of this approach is that it combines openness and also boundaries for privacy—each couple gets to decide what to go public about, and within that zone of privacy there is permission to probe, support, and challenge. Once this small community of five couples is solid, they plan to expand and create a larger, intentional community.

• Hold public rituals. These could be planned by the cluster groups and coordinated by staff members of the organization. I suggest three kinds of public rituals for marriage: anniversary rituals, healing rituals, and reconciliation rituals. These probably fit best in a religious community where they can express the spirituality of a particular congregation.

• I have wanted for years to come up with a practical new approach to getting support for couples in their own life worlds. Now I have developed "The Marital First Responders Project," a way to train people who are natural confidants to be even more helpful when family members and friends reach out to talk about problems in their marriage. These supportive people are everywhere; they are caring and good listeners. In fact, they are the first responders to marital crises because they have relationships of trust with other people. The project trains them to be even more capable of making a difference for others' marriages, avoiding common pitfalls (like taking sides prematurely), and knowing what good sources of help to steer their friends to. You can learn about this project at *www. maritalfirstresponders.com.*

When it comes to supporting marriages in communities, especially faith communities, I have been struck by the importance of holding on to two important truths about marriage. On the one hand, marriage is a wonderful spiritual and physical bond between two human beings, and a central undergirding for human community. On the other hand, it is a flawed human relationship between two limited people who struggle against powerful forces to make their love last. Faith communities that celebrate the glories of marriage without making space for its dark side will drive many couples underground to lick their wounds in secrecy and shame. Even faith communities that have made good strides in recognizing and responding to the suffering of those whose marriages have ended are slow to recognize the same need in those who are struggling to make their imperfect marriage work.

Once, during a workshop I gave for therapists on taking a pro-commitment stand in therapy, a woman approached to tell me about her response to her daughter's sudden announcement that she and her husband were going to divorce. The mother was a therapist trained to be "neutral" about divorce and to believe that parents should not meddle in the life choices of their adult children. But she was feeling decidedly not neutral about her daughter ending a marriage with young children without seeking help to salvage it. When her daughter said, "Mom, I am going to get a divorce," the mother blurted out: "Over my dead body you will! You are going to get into therapy before you make any decision, and I will help you find a good therapist." The daughter, taken aback, agreed. With tearful eyes, the mother told me that her daughter's marriage was still alive and now prospering. Instead of feeling embarrassed at her outburst, the mother now felt proud of it.

Solitary marriage fits well with today's consumer culture of marriage, but it is lonely and fragile. When the cold and rain come, we need the shelter of more than each other, knowing that a promarriage community will not only nurture us but also make demands on us as citizens to take our marital commitment seriously and to be stakeholders in the marriages of others around us. We either stand together for marriages in our communities, or else we will be picked off one by one, the weakest first, by a culture that preys on long-term love. Even if you feel strong in your marriage, consider that the next weak one in the pack might be your friend's marriage, or your daughter's. We have to build a world that is safe for marriage.

12 Taking Action for Your Marriage

If you have stayed with me this long, you may be convinced that you have to keep taking your marriage back from the me-first consumer culture and from the natural drift south of your marital canoe. There is no resting on laurels in today's marriages. You also may be convinced that you want your marriage to be intentional, committed-no-matter-what, and community based. This isn't a 1970s version of the "self-actualized" couple; this is about marital survival in today's world.

We've been talking about action steps all along, so why an extra discussion of "taking action for your marriage"? For starters, you are probably reading this book by yourself; your spouse or partner, if you have one, probably has not been reading it over your shoulder. This creates dangers and opportunities if you decide to use what you have learned here.

Why This Book Can Be Dangerous to Your Marriage—and How to Make It Good for Your Marriage

Every marital therapist has seen it, I've done it myself, and perhaps you have too, if you are the kind of person who reads books like this one. You feel the thrill of new information and insight, or perhaps the strong affirmation of a piece of important wisdom you already had. "This is really going to help my marriage," you say to yourself.

Given our self-absorbed natures (I'll speak for myself at least), we assume in our hearts that our mate really needs this new perspective even more than we do ourselves. After all, if you are the one who scours books and articles for new ideas for your marriage, aren't you the hunter for a better relationship?

From here the scenario can go one of two ways. While you are devouring the book, you gush to your mate that he or she simply *must* read it as soon as you are finished. Now maybe you and your spouse are used to freely trading books on relationships, in which case you are free and clear; your spouse will read it and form an independent judgment on its usefulness. I know there are couples like that out there; it's just that I have only met a few, usually one in each state I have lived in. By the way, my wife and I are not in this group. We are more like the next group.

The second direction of the scenario goes like this: you gush over the *great* ideas in this new book, and your mate wonders what changes you are cooking up for the relationship. What new fish are you about to bring home to clean and cook? Your spouse remembers the last time you got enthusiastic about a change in your sex life, and the sprained back that ensued.

How would this second scenario look after you finish this book? You are fired up about, say, having more and better marital rituals, or about getting more connected with a community of couples. Undeniably wonderful ideas, if you ask me. If your spouse had come across these ideas separately, without your well-intended efforts at education, he or she might feel the same way. (That's why I like to give talks and workshops for couples, not individual spouses, and to work with couples in therapy. They are both hearing the message at the same time, and can each like it or not, without as much pressure from the other. With books, I cannot assume two independent readers in the same marriage.)

When you propose a change in your marital relationship, you almost inevitably come across as saying that something is wrong or deficient in the status quo. If I were your spouse, maybe I would think we were doing just fine, thank you, and tell you so. Whereupon you would try to impress on me the view that things are not so great that they can't be improved upon. "We need better rituals, better ways for us to connect," you'd say. "First of all," I'd retort, "our religious rituals are just fine, and we connect better than most couples I know." Now you get to the dirty truth: "You know, I've been wanting to connect more with you, but you are so stuck in your ways. I'm always the one trying to make things better for us, and you fight me."

I will spare you the rest of the scene. Call it Act II, Scene 33, of this couple's pursuer–distancer dance. And for this outcome you paid good money for this book!

You no doubt get my point. New ideas coming from one spouse can disturb the balance of a marriage. Adding new patterns to an established marriage is like changing dance steps while holding each other during the middle of a tune. It is certainly not impossible—couples do it all the time—but it requires, shall we say, a degree of finesse, especially if you do not have a history of making intentional changes to your relationship. If your previous suggestions came across as criticism, then you especially have to watch your step. If you find it hard to change well-entrenched habits of relating, you are not alone.

Here is a range of ways to approach your mate about implementing the ideas in this book. I will arrange them from most indirect to most direct, keeping in mind that no approach is the "correct" one. (Indirect approaches, for example, may work better in your marriage than direct ones.) The first approach is really a matter of discovering what you are already doing, and being conscious about it. The rest are ways to introduce new behavior.

• Notice something connecting that you are already doing together and say that you would like to make it a regular ritual in your marriage. This works especially well for elevating a marital routine into a ritual. When my wife and I evolved a postdinner coffee conversation, we didn't think of its importance at first. But at some point, we referred to it as "our coffee time" and became conscious of its importance to us. We had turned a routine into a ritual, which meant that we were committed to it and it helped to define our marriage. Naming a marital ritual is a simple but powerful way to change your relationship. The key is to solicit an agreement to make this activity a regular part of your life, and to protect it.

• Make something new happen without advance comment. For example, if you haven't dated in a long time, check the calendar, get a sitter, make the reservations, and announce to your spouse that you are inviting him or her out on a special date. Do your best to make it a lovely time, and at the end, if you sense your mate has enjoyed it too, suggest that the two of you do this regularly. If your spouse is willing, then negotiate the specifics of the ritual you want to put into place—frequency, types of dates, responsibility, and logistics. The advantage of this approach is that the two of you make the decision to change after you have experienced the new activity. You act first and then talk about more permanent change. This approach is particularly useful if you and your spouse tend to get bogged down when you talk about making changes.

• Bring up a new idea tentatively. I call this the "Minnesota Shuffle." It's especially useful if you are like me, someone known for coming across too strongly about new ideas. You say something like, "I was thinking that maybe we could try something different at bedtime. It may not work because I get tired before you do, and I know that you enjoy your time alone in the evening. I don't know if it's worth thinking about trying something different." You wait for an invitation from your spouse, such as "What do you have in mind?" Whereupon you reply that you are thinking about just a small thing instead of changing your whole nighttime routine. Wait for another invitation, verbal or nonverbal. Then make your proposal, say, for a good-night cuddle before you go to sleep. If this approach would feel manipulative to you, then don't use it. I think of it not as manipulative but as tentatively testing the waters to see whether your spouse is open to a conversation on the topic before you waste your new idea at the wrong moment.

• Bring up your need but without a solution at this point. You can plant seeds for future change by saying how you feel about something, and what you need, without prescribing a particular solution or blaming your mate for the current situation. In the date example, you can say, during a calm time, that you miss going out as a couple and wish there was a way to put that back in your marriage. If you can predict, based on experience, that your spouse will respond with a volley of logistical and other obstacles (probably all of them accurate and ones that you have raised yourself), then just repeat your feelings and say that some time in the future, you hope it might be possible to overcome the obstacles and enjoy each other on dates. Don't say much more. Don't argue about implementation. Just let your need and desire float for a while in your relationship before you bring up the subject again for action. Your spouse will know it's on your mind. In the bedtime example, you can simply say that you miss having contact before you go to sleep, but that you realize it's nobody's fault. When you make a proposal in the future, it will build upon this prior conversation.

• Bring up a need and an idea for change, but do not push for a decision. As before, always start with something you need or believe the relationship needs, as opposed to starting with the solution. This grounds the conversation in something other than your willfulness or wish to tinker with the relationship. Always ask your spouse what he or she needs too, but don't challenge your spouse about not needing something as much as you do. (That's a lost cause.) Sometimes, when you have thought through a new plan of action, your mate may need some time to see its merits. And of course, with time to reflect, your spouse might improve upon it and come up with a better alternative. This approach involves floating the idea but saying up front that you are not looking for a decision right now. It's just something to think about, like the notion of building a new patio for the house some day. If your spouse responds favorably, so much the better. But if he or she responds with a volley of objections, you can say, "Let's just think about it. Maybe something else will work better. I just wanted to plant the idea." And back out of the conversation if it is turning into an argument. Your spouse will think about it further, as will you.

• Bring up a need and a specific idea for a decision and a trial run. This approach often works best if you have broached the topic before, in ways such as those above. Here you are saying that you would like to do something different, want to hear your mate's feelings and perspectives, and then make a decision. You do have a particular change in mind, such as biweekly dates or a cuddle at bedtime. If you are truly negotiating, you must be open to modifying your plan, to hearing objections you had not considered, and to trying a different approach toward the same goal. But you are letting your spouse know that you want to do something different. It's a good idea, though, to frame the change as an experiment that you will both learn from. How will the bedtime cuddle actually work in practice? How will it have to be modified? Proposing an experiment that you will both evaluate keeps you from assuming the power position of dictating the future of your relationship.

• Bring up the big picture of your relationship and your desire for change. Broach your feelings about how your relationship is going and your wish for general change, but don't tie it to any specific change, and especially not a unilateral change by your spouse. Rehearse how you bring this up, because it won't be easy. Do it at a calm time and be prepared to be empathetic to your mate's feelings and fears about what you are trying to do here. You are acting as a marital citizen and leader. This might be a conversation where you call for a more intentional marriage, a more conscious, planful, and mutual approach to growing your relationship because you feel your marriage drifting. Your spouse is likely to want to focus on your specific complaints, especially if this conversation is a surprise, but don't get lost in details. If this book, or another, has been influential in how you are thinking about what you want in your marriage, then tell your spouse that, for the purpose of full disclosure. Offer to share it if your spouse is interested, but don't push it, lest the book itself become the source of a power struggle. Reaffirm your love and your commitment-no-matter-what, and walk sensitively and without blame into the uncharted waters of substantial change in your marriage. Because your larger agenda and set of needs are now out on the table, your mate might be motivated to respond more openly when you bring up specific ideas in the future. Of course, maybe not. I used this approach a number of years ago when I raised a concern that we were not as intentional about our financial future as we were about other aspects of our marriage. Leah at first thought I was suggesting that we were not being responsible with our specific financial decisions (like what we purchase), but came to see that my concern was different: it was about our overall financial planning for the future. We eventually decided we needed outside help to be more intentional about this part of our lives, and began to work with a good financial planner.

• Bring up the idea of getting help to move your marriage onto a new course. If the approaches I described above get you nowhere, then it may be that right now neither you nor your spouse can exercise the kind of marital leadership that is required for change. You are stuck on the river and can't agree on a plan for paddling. The first place to turn would be to a marriage education activity in your faith community or wider community. A good listing of what is available in different parts of the country is available from the Coalition of Marriage, Family and Couple Education at *smartmarriages. com*. In marriage education, you can learn together new ways to take charge of your marital journey. You can develop your relationship skills, and you can be around other couples who are intentional about their marriages. The second place to turn, if marriage education is not available or not sufficient, is marital therapy. See our earlier discussion about what to avoid and what to seek in a marital therapist who can help you jump-start your marriage again.

And the Wisdom to Know the Difference

This has been a book about making changes, about being proactive, about taking charge of your marriage's future in an unfriendly world. I want to end with words about the importance of accepting what will not change. Every marriage has two people who have what psychologist William Bradbury calls "enduring vulnerabilities." These are personal qualities from our backgrounds that limit us as individuals and marriage partners, and that cause pain or frustration for us and those we love. Maybe it was the experience of our parents' divorce that makes us cling so tightly to our mate that it's hard for that person to breathe. Maybe it's a bit of attention-deficit/hyperactivity disorder that makes it hard to settle into predictable marital rituals. Maybe a critical family left us supersensitive to criticism or too eager to dish it out. The possibilities are as endless as they are real in our lives. For the most part, they are not going to go away.

Some of these vulnerabilities are clear before we marry someone, but many are not. It takes the furnace of marital intimacy to bring them forth. That's partly why every marriage is a surprise to its inhabitants. But over time many of us learn to accept and cope well with our vulnerabilities and those of our spouse, and to offset each other's weaknesses. We come to realize that if we ditch this spouse for someone else, we are in for another surprise, and maybe a nastier one, that we will have to learn to cope with all over again.

Add to our personal vulnerabilities the way that we teach boys and girls to be different and then expect them to be happy, well-adjusted life mates. For most of us, our experience of marriage is never going to match our original expectations and desires. Some of us will never get the kind of emotional attention we thought we would get when we found our soul mate. Others of us will never have the kind of comfortable, low-maintenance relationship we thought we would get when we married a person we felt so easy to be with. We can learn to adjust, but certain problematic differences endure.

Accepting less than what we want goes against the grain of the consumer culture of entitlement. Lifelong marriage means accepting who we both are and forsaking new, improved models of a husband or wife—again, not what the marketplace teaches. Commitment-no-matter-what means that I am faithful to a flawed human being, who is faithful to me as a flawed human being, in a moral covenant that does not have a lemon clause and does not permit leasing and trade-ins, with tragic exceptions, of course. And it means we never stop working on being married.

I once heard a radio interview with a beloved figure in my home state of Minnesota, the former Governor Elmer Andersen, then age ninety, who had just written a memoir about his life and career in a wide range of public service activities. He has been married for sixty-eight years. When asked the perennial "what's your secret?" question, he gave a most unusual and profound answer: "We are still getting accustomed to being married."

This commitment to never stop working on our marriage, combined with acceptance of each other's limitations, means that we can feel safe enough to battle with each other at times about the direction of our canoe. It allows us to say, "I'm in this marriage boat for good, baby, and I'm not interested in the Gulf of Mexico. I say we pick up our paddles, exercise some muscles that have weakened through lack of use, and head north again. And along the way, let's gather ourselves a convoy and take St. Paul by storm."

Index

P

Parent–child rituals, 21–22. *See also* Rituals of connection and intimacy

Parenting. *See also* Children-first approach to marriage; Intentional parenting; Parent–child rituals
changing and how children will react to, 60–61
consumer culture and, 36–38
intentional marriage and, 21–22
marriage-centered family and, 64–66
not losing your marriage to, 62–64
overscheduling issues and, 72–73
stepfamily situations and, 86–89

Parents of you or your spouse. *See also* Family of origin
expectations regarding marriage and, 95–97
undermining of your marriage and, 81–86

Pathology, marital therapy and, 106–107

Permeance. *See also* Commitment
consumer marriage and, 31–34
overview, 24
value of life-long commitment, 4–8

Previous marriages, 86–89

Privilege, marriage as, 4

Public rituals, 178–179. *See also* Rituals of connection and intimacy

Pursuer–distancer cycle. *See also* Time for your marriage
marital rituals and, 143
normalcy of, 172
overscheduling issues and, 72–73
overview, 67–68
reclaiming time for your marriage and, 79

R

Reconciliation rituals, 179. *See also* Rituals of connection and intimacy

Recreation
single friends and, 89–90
time for your marriage and, 73–75, 79

Remarriage, 86–89. *See also* Stepfamilies

"Renewable marriage," 31

Renewal, marital. *See* Marital renewal

Renewal, vision of. *See* Vision of renewal

Resistance to outside forces, 25–26. *See also* Intentional marriage; Marital renewal

Responsibilities
consumer culture and, 36–38
divorce and, 41–43

Righteousness, consumer marriage and, 50–51

Rituals in families, 57–59

Rituals of connection and intimacy. *See also* Anniversaries; Connection rituals; Courtship rituals; Intimacy rituals; Love rituals; Marital rituals; Parent–child rituals; Special occassions; Talk rituals
bedtimes and, 57–59
changes in, 181–189
children-first approach to marriage and, 62–63
creativity of, 144–146, 166–167
intentional marriage and, 20–22
overview, 19–20, 137–140

S

Satisfaction in marriage, 16–19. *See also* Dissatisfaction in marriage; Happiness in marriage

Schedules. *See also* Time for your marriage
overscheduling issues and, 72–73
reclaiming time for your marriage and, 78–80

About the Author

William J. Doherty, PhD, is Professor and Director of the Minnesota Couples on the Brink Project at the University of Minnesota, and a practicing marriage and family therapist. Past president of the National Council on Family Relations, he received the Council's Margaret E. Arcus Award for Outstanding Contribution to Family Life Education. Dr. Doherty is the author of numerous books for professionals and general readers. Married since 1971, he has two grown children and four grandchildren.